I0424108

God's Grand Design for Health

JAMES DARNELL, D.C.

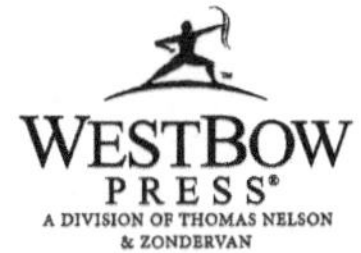

WestBow Press books may be ordered through booksellers or by contacting:

WestBow Press
A Division of Thomas Nelson & Zondervan
1663 Liberty Drive
Bloomington, IN 47403
www.westbowpress.com
1 (866) 928-1240

ISBN: 978-1-5127-8641-5 (sc)
ISBN: 978-1-5127-8640-8 (hc)
ISBN: 978-1-5127-8642-2 (e)

Library of Congress Control Number: 2017906814

Print information available on the last page.

WestBow Press rev. date: 07/26/2017

CONTENTS

FOREWORD

You, the reader, are about to embark on a journey through a quarter century of consummate research and clinical application that's been proven to help people regain optimal function. The author's application of that knowledge has resulted in countless miracles and saved lives!

Having a foundational philosophy that we are all energy is of paramount importance in understanding the true origins of health. The author owns and lives that truth and eloquently shares it for the benefit of you and your loved ones in the pages that follow.

In order to truly shift our paradigm in health care, we must start with the fact that we are spirit first, mind second and body last. The body-mind-spirit adage needs to be stood on its head, and the truths in these pages do just that.

While this book emphasizes proper nutrition and the toxins to which we are exposed, it most importantly has the necessary foundational understanding of acid-alkaline pH balance. It will teach you the primary disruptors of that delicate pH balance and the impact on the cells if that balance is disrupted.

This brilliant compilation of golden nuggets of truth in the arena of proper nutrition starts with a frank, eye-opening look at where the United States stands as a nation in health care. World Health Organization statistics for 2015 shows the US ranking thirty-fourth among all industrialized nations in life expectancy. The United States Central Intelligence Agency shows US life expectancy ranked at forty-second in life expectancy for 2016, reflecting a less than stellar grade in the performance of our health-care system. If forty-one countries are doing a better job at healthcare, something is grossly missing in our approach. Our nation is literally dying to hear the truths that are revealed in the pages of this book.

Prepare to have your paradigm shifted. You, the reader, will anxiously await this book's sequel, as I do, to further enlighten us about better health, optimizing our lives.

—Kreg D. Huffer DC LCP

PREFACE

> The illiterate of the 21st century will not be those who cannot read or write but those who cannot learn, unlearn, and relearn.
>
> —Alvin Toffler

The contents of this book are a summary of things I have learned over the course of a twenty-three-year career as a practicing chiropractic physician. This book would have looked completely different if it was written even ten years ago. Life is a journey, and we are all on a path of learning and evolving with our newfound knowledge. My hope is that you, the reader, will find tidbits of knowledge that you can use on your journey as well.

I could not complete this book without giving credit to the many influences I have had along the way. Among them are my friend and mentor Dr. Kreg Huffer, whose friendship and guidance have kept me on the correct path more times than I care to mention, and my wife, Sheryl, whose love and support through the writing process has made this all possible.

And finally, to the many colleagues and instructors who have influenced my life in a positive way, a big thank-you. Two in particular, Dr. Dan Murphy and Dr. Brandon Lundell, unknowingly inspired me to press forward with my research and desire to write this book. It is extremely difficult to sit in seminar after seminar, seeing all this data flash before me, knowing that our society is not receiving the message. Yes, I can and do talk to patients in my office, but that is such a limited sphere of influence. To get the word out to the masses, I realized more needs to be done even if it means spending an entire year researching, compiling data, and putting it all in print.

My training as a chiropractor is heavily weighted in prevention of disease rather than curing illness. In fact, it is woven through every fabric of my being. It's not just something I do; it's part of who I am. Prevention is a core premise of chiropractic as well as other holistic professions like acupuncture, homeopathy, and naturopathy.

My primary goal of writing this book is to raise awareness of the need for a preventive lifestyle and preventive health care. As the rate of chronic disease continues to escalate, the health-care picture becomes cloudier and cloudier. Statistics indicate that more Americans are becoming interested in prevention and are more inclined than ever before to buy supplements and natural products. Even in my clinical practice I have noticed a similar trend with many of my patients. However, there are still patients who have resisted active measures of prevention, even after attending health orientation classes in my office and seeing the importance of it firsthand.

The common resistance is "you have to die sometime. Why should I waste my time and money on supplements and adjustments if it's not going to change the outcome?" To me the answer is simple. The Bible says in the book of Ecclesiastes, "To everything there is a season, and a time for every purpose under heaven." This includes "a time to be born and a time to die." They are right in their argument to a certain extent. The deeper issue is quality of life. Jesus says in The Gospel of John, "The thief comes only to steal and kill and destroy; I have come that they may have life, and have it to the full." John 10:10 (NIV) It's difficult to have a full, abundant life when you're battling a chronic illness. God can work out his purpose for your life even in the presence of illness, but it's much easier to take care of the temple with preventive measures now, so we can enjoy the benefits of it and be a light for his glory. So, on a deeper level, getting started and sustaining new habits seems to be a major hurdle for some people.

What comes to mind when you think of preventive health care? The younger generations will more than likely associate preventive health care with some form of technology. After all, the gold standard for health care in America involves advancements in medical technology. Mammography, MRIs, CT scans, and high-tech pharmaceuticals and vaccines are on the cutting edge of medical advancements. While these are all very positive improvements, when I step back and look at the big picture of twenty-first-century health care, I see a picture that has carried us away from the foundation of where health truly begins. A mammogram can detect a tumor in the breast, but it does not address the factors that created the tumor. It has even been suggested that mammography leads to overdiagnosis and overtreatment.[1]

The same is true with MRI and CT scans. They can see tumors and other pathological changes inside the body, but they don't address the factors that created the pathology. High-tech pharmaceuticals can target tumors, regulate blood pressure, suppress an overactive immune system, and provide therapies for just about any condition. But every one of these interventions implies that the body is already broken. What about addressing the factors that create the broken body in the first place before they become pathological? Where does prevention fit in twenty-first-century health care? Vaccines can *prevent* the onset of many infectious diseases, but even this method of prevention comes at a high cost to those who are vaccinated. Allergies, autism, and autoimmune disorders are just a few of the documented secondary effects of vaccinations that frequently show up later in life. These issues and many others reveal the shortcomings of relying exclusively on the technology model of health care.

Can true prevention of disease really be achieved in the twenty-first century? I emphatically say yes. Yes, it can be done. I've seen it in my practice with my own eyes. The caveat is I don't think we can get there exclusively through the technology model. In fact I'm convinced of it. Natural forms of prevention like proper diet and nutrition are the very foundation of health, which we seem to have lost sight of in our fast-paced modern lives. Proper diet and nutritional supplementation can be very effective in preventing disease if used properly. Yet this seems to be in indirect opposition to where a large portion of our culture seems to be heading.

I am boldly suggesting that our approach to health care needs to be modified if we are going to address the true underlying cause of the diseases of the twenty-first century. We have to get back to basics, starting with proper diet and working our way down the list of preventive measures, such as exercise, stress reduction, and taking time to smell the roses. As we reorganize our priorities, we can begin by slowing down the pace of our lives so that eating quality foods and exercising becomes an achievable goal. We hear about dental hygiene from the dentists—cleanings twice a year to prevent cavities. The spine is the control center of the body. What about proper spinal hygiene through regular chiropractic care? What about connecting with our creator through prayer and meditation? These things *are* enough to create a significant change in the health of our culture. The question is can we get there in our fast-paced society?

I have had the good fortune to learn from very intelligent people who are not afraid to challenge the existing reality. These great minds are the catalysts that sparked my desire to learn. We can learn lessons from our experiences, as well as from the experiences of other people. There is value in taking a long, hard look at where you've been, where you're at, and where you're headed. A good dose of objective reality can keep you heading in the right direction (as long as you don't get stuck there). Knowledge is power; sharing that knowledge is even more powerful.

The pages that follow are full of facts that give a true picture of where we, as a nation, stand on health care. It's an alarming picture of where we are heading if we don't change course. If this book does not present an overwhelming case for a change in direction, I don't know what will. The data is not provided to overwhelm you; rather it is provided to get your attention.

Why? Because if more people understood these concepts, there is no question in my mind we would have a healthier society. The only way that will happen is if more people start writing about it and educating all who will listen.

INTRODUCTION

> Give a man a fish, he eats for a day; teach a man to fish, he eats for a lifetime.
>
> —Anne Ritchie

Making healthier choices is an empowering process, a process that involves knowing what things to avoid that can cause illness, as well as knowing what things should be part of your life that will enhance your health. Where do you start?

Building a house requires a blueprint. Traveling to an unfamiliar destination requires a map. Being healthy and staying healthy are no different. The caveat in the discussion of health is that "the blueprint" is more complicated. It's not a straight line. It involves a large number of variables. One thing is certain: it is hard to live to your full potential if you're not healthy. That's why living a healthy lifestyle should be everyone's number one priority. It's easy to let other things take higher priority until you experience a health crisis. A health crisis has a unique way of reorganizing priorities. I have seen this scenario many times during my twenty-three years of practice. People often take their health for granted until some form of crisis strikes. For some, the first crisis is severe, such as a heart attack or a cancer diagnosis. Will you be included in that life-changing statistic?

What does living to your full potential mean to you? For most people, it probably means having a good job, a nice home, and a family. For some it means becoming the next great scientist, maybe even the future president of the United States. I hope living healthy is included somewhere in those lofty goals.

I firmly believe with knowledge comes wisdom. Knowledge is worthless if it is not shared. Teaching and sharing information has always been a central theme of my practice. As time has passed, teaching has become even more critical. Why? As a nation we are slowly getting sicker and suffering from chronic diseases at younger ages. There is a wealth of great information available on health and wellness topics in print and on television.

As my colleague Dr. Dan Murphy says, "The people who have published some of this information are really smart dudes."

From my perspective, he's right. Never in the history of humankind have we understood so much about health. If that is true, why are we still experiencing an explosion of chronic illness? Is it because the information is still only reaching a limited audience? Is it because the information is too complicated and needs to be simplified? Is it because people are busy trying to survive? Perhaps it is all the above. I think these are just a few of the challenges to the future health of humankind—taking the time to learn new habits and discard old ones that have been proven to be false, then applying that information to everyday life in a practical way. It's easy to read a new book on diet or exercise and get excited that you have learned something new. Applying that new information and sustaining it in our daily lives is where it becomes more difficult. Sometimes it takes a reorganization of priorities to make it happen. Mere survival can easily crowd out health-enhancing habits.

I have learned that people don't know what they don't know and what they don't know causes them to make poor choices that lead to poor health. This is compounded by the paradoxical fact that we make decisions based on what we already know, which often limits our ability to learn new information. The road to health does not happen by chance. It requires specific action steps from all of us. Too many people leave it to chance, which is like playing Russian roulette with their most prized possession, their health.

The core of my training as a chiropractic physician is centered on the vitalistic concept of preventing disease rather than curing illness. This concept is woven into every fabric of my being. (My wife and others who know me can attest to this fact.) It becomes a way of life that you live rather than just something that you do.

Where does prevention fit in this discussion? There is tremendous value in preventive methods, whether it is improving your diet, getting your spine adjusted, exercising, or finding better ways to handle stress. Each of these items are within our control, but all too often I encounter people who feel somewhat out of control in these areas as if life is leading them instead of them leading their lives. As author Steven Covey writes, taking charge of your life begins with developing a healthy paradigm and then being proactive about your choices[2]. I believe most people don't realize how big the impact will be from simple lifestyle changes. I can't begin to tell you how many patients have said to me after they start receiving chiropractic care, "I didn't realize how bad I felt until I started to feel better. I just accepted that (you name the symptoms) will always be there." Major improvements can come from the simplest things.

When we focus on prevention, the reward for everyone becomes better health and less sickness. As the Bible says, "Whatever a man sows, he shall also reap" Galatians 6:7 (NKJV). We must start teaching people how to sow better seeds, meaning how to live healthier lives. As individuals we reap better health. As a nation we lower health-care costs. Everyone wins.

Limited Paradigm vs. Proactive Habits

I believe that much of what we do is truly out of habit. "This is just the way I've always done it" is a common theme that I hear. Habits are a strong motivator; old habits are hard to break. Developing a healthier lifestyle takes time and effort, but it's always worth it. And there is never a more important topic than learning about things that keep us healthy and things that make us sick. Health care, or caring for one's health, must become a lifestyle that is more than a visit to the doctor. Health care should begin when you go to the grocery store and choose your foods. Stress management—through prayer, meditation, and exercise—is very important for good health. Cleansing your body of toxins is important too. Chiropractic adjustments will keep the frame of the body in proper alignment and remove interference from the nervous system, which leads to pain and illness. The people who have experienced the benefits of these things will tell you how valuable they are in their lives. Why are these habits not a regular part of our society?

Sorting Out Fact From Fiction

> You never change things by fighting the existing reality. True, lasting change builds a new model that makes the old model obsolete.
>
> —Buckminster Fuller

We live in an information age where a wealth of knowledge is at our fingertips. Some of it is true; some of it is not. Still, information forces us to prioritize our time and what we allow into our brain.

Author Buckminster Fuller made an interesting observation. Looking back over history, Fuller noticed that until the year 1900, human knowledge seemed to double approximately every century. By the end of World War II, human knowledge was accelerating, doubling every twenty-five years. At our present rate, it is estimated that human knowledge is doubling every thirteen months. Oh, but here's the rub. How do you sort out fact from fiction? What topics deserve the majority of your precious time?

How you answer these questions depends on your background, your beliefs, and your values. All information that enters your brain is filtered through these basic elements that form your paradigm. We evaluate new information based on what we already know. In terms of human psychology and motivation, new information that enters your brain is challenged, accepted, or rejected. It has been this way since the beginning of time. We form beliefs from this information. This becomes our paradigm, our unique way of seeing the world around us. A false perception of reality does not change the truth even if a large number of people believe it to be true.

As you read further, you'll see examples of false perceptions which had to be discarded for the greater progress of humankind. This is good! We all have some outdated paradigms tucked somewhere in our brain. I hope you're like me; I want to fill my mind with the right things and not let the world dictate those things for me.

Throughout my years in practice, I have often been reminded how entrenched certain belief systems have become related to health and well-being. Beliefs influence people's decisions in a profound way but especially when related to health and disease. This disease runs in my family. Both of my parents died in their 50's so I probably will as well. No, we're not just sitting ducks, waiting for disease to strike. Disease prevention is a lifestyle that filters down through the choices we make.

However prevalent and popular they become, beliefs are not always based on valid, factual information. Change is often difficult. Old beliefs die slowly. History proves it. Here are some thoughts as to why.

As I observe what is happening in our society, it is apparent to me that the volume of information regarding health and wellness has become overwhelming to most people, even doctors. As a physician, there is simply not enough time in the day to read every relevant piece of literature. Finding the time to communicate information to patients on a busy day is a real challenge. The content of your communication matters too. I have learned it is better to communicate small amounts of quality information than a large amount of information that will soon be forgotten. Even then, how do physicians prioritize what information should be communicated? That is a relevant and important question.

The latest edition of the Physicians' Desk Reference (PDR), long considered the holy grail of pharmaceutical information, is 2000 pages. Talk about information overload! Physicians and consumers alike must choose what information enters our minds. Even then, the brain only retains a limited amount of that information, so choose wisely.

Aside from the sheer volume, much of the information out there can become very complicated. Simplifying that information to understandable components is something we all must do at one time or another. For most people, if something is too complicated, it seems to fall by the wayside.

Complicated information can generate a cynical attitude even when it involves an important topic like finding a new approach to staying healthy. "How do I fit that into my schedule?" is the common resistance I hear. And they're right. Every day in my practice I see families who are overly busy and exhausted taking care of the kids and holding down full-time jobs. Finding time for healthy habits is almost an afterthought. There is little time left to devote to important things, such as planning proper meals, exercising, sleeping, prayer, meditation, and all the other little things that go into keeping us healthy. And that just touches the surface of it all.

You say, "I'll go to the bookstore and read books on health and wellness." That's a great idea. But stroll through the bookstore and you'll quickly realize just how vast the choices and opinions are related to health topics. Where do you start? Even a simple topic like what you should eat has evolved into a complex subject:

- Should I eat a high-protein diet?
- Maybe I should eat a low-fat diet with higher portions of carbohydrates.
- Wait. Didn't I read that carbohydrates are bad for you?
- Wait. Carbohydrates are only bad for people of certain blood types.
- Oh yeah, and high-protein diets are hard on the kidneys, right?

See what I mean? A healthy diet is no longer just meat and potatoes. Opinions on diet have become so numerous that it's easy to get overwhelmed by your choices. And diet is only one factor in the health discussion. No wonder people are getting lost in a sea of information.

As life becomes busier and more complex, I am concerned people will continue to make choices that will lead them down the wrong path. We are already seeing this on a broad scale in our country. As I said, people don't know what they don't know. It's more involved. They also don't know what they need to know. It's pretty tough to get where you need to go if you don't know your destination.

There must be a way to simplify things; otherwise, people quickly return to old habits. The old adage is true: If you always do as you've always done, you will get what you've always gotten. Don't be one of those people.

Health Tip: The path to any chronic illness is a process, not an event.

Like a seed that is planted in the ground, chronic illness takes time to develop. You don't simply wake up one day and find yourself unhealthy. A healthy body is something that must be nurtured like a garden. Unfortunately, many of us are planting the wrong seeds and failing to nurture the garden (our bodies). Some are doing so unknowingly. What a tragedy. Don't let this happen to you.

Of the thousands of people I have encountered in my career, I have not encountered one person who wants to be unhealthy. Not one. I have encountered many who simply didn't know how to live a preventive lifestyle. Yes, there are some who are unwilling to put in the work necessary to stay healthy, but the vast majority of people are willing if they are shown how to do it. Prevention doesn't come without a price. Preventing illness requires an extra degree of personal responsibility. We are not just passive observers without any control over our health. This is the fallacy of believing you are just a product of your genes. Believing this is a step toward giving up your power to make better choices in order to improve your health. Focus on the things you can change, and leave the results to the almighty. That's the solution to sanity and lasting change.

I'm convinced that improving the health of our nation begins with three things: (1) changing our beliefs about preventive health care, (2) learning how toxins affect the body, and (3) improving our dietary habits. The starting point for disease prevention is learning how toxins affect our bodies. From there we can learn how to protect ourselves from toxic overload. It all begins with a proper diet.

As you read this information, keep in mind this is not presented as a diagnosis or cure for any disease process. It is simply presented to get you to think about wellness as a lifestyle and to create awareness about how disease develops in the body. We certainly know much more now than we did even ten or twenty years ago. The responsibility for that awareness and making lifestyle changes begins with each of us as individuals. As you become more aware of the things you are doing wrong, it is easier to make appropriate changes. God helps those who help themselves.

In my own life, God as often directed me to the resources and people I needed at exactly the right time. This led me to realize we are co-creators of our lives and not just innocent bystanders. That is my vision for the information I'm giving you in this book. If we do all that we can do, God will do the things we can't do on our own. This includes helping us stay healthy.

CHAPTER 1

Health: Where Are We and Where Are We Heading?

> I desire to know why one person was ailing and his associate, eating at the same table, working in the same shop, at the same bench, was not. Why? What difference was there in these two persons that caused one to have various diseases, while his partner escaped?
>
> —D. D. Palmer
> founder of the chiropractic profession

Over the years, I've often asked myself this question: Why do some people get sick and some don't?

Here's another challenging question: Is it possible to live a vibrantly healthy life from birth until death? I'm not talking about occasionally contracting the common cold or flu. I'm talking about as a culture living healthfully and avoiding debilitating illnesses until we reach the century mark or death at a ripe old age. It seems a bit paradoxical to think that there are more centenarians now in America than ever before and yet so many younger Americans are developing debilitating illnesses by the time they reach their forties. Something is wrong with that picture.

The notion of living to a ripe old age and just stepping off the earth when your days are finished seems quite appealing to me, especially when you've witnessed loved ones dying slow, painful deaths from some disease or affliction. So is it possible to live to be a healthy centenarian in this modern age? Do beliefs and expectations have any bearing on that longevity? Before you say no, consider this:

In some cultures, living well beyond one hundred years is the expectation. Many years ago I read an article from *National Geographic* magazine that profoundly shaped my thinking on the longevity issue. The article, "Every Day Is a Gift When You're Over 100," was an investigative report on the life of the Hunza tribe in the southern Himalayan mountains.[3]

For those of you who are unfamiliar with the Hunzas, the article says these tribal people routinely live well into their hundreds. Disease as we know it in our society is pretty much nonexistent for them. In fact, they have a requirement that anyone on the city council must be at least one hundred years of age. Anyone younger than that simply hasn't lived long enough to have the wisdom required for city council. The centenarians are out in the fields harvesting crops right along with the fifty-year-olds.

Just how long do these people actually live? One of the article's primary sources was a lady who estimated her age to be 144 years. She had to estimate her age because no official records were kept when she was born. Her account of her age was based on historical events (e.g., she was ten years old when such and such event happened). She also claimed to have had a pack-a-day smoking habit since she was in her teens.

The oldest member of the tribe was estimated to be 167 years old. At the time the article was published, that would mean he was alive when Abraham Lincoln was president. That gets my attention! It makes me wonder, how do they live that long?

A key part of the article talked about the decline in health when certain members were taken from the tribe to live in the city. Within a short time, the transplanted tribal members developed sicknesses much like we have in our society. That is a significant clue for all of us who have never experienced other cultures. At home their food was naturally grown with no chemicals. Stress was nonexistent, and there was no theft or violence. They also believed what's mine is yours and yours is mine. These were the keys to their longevity. But while living in the city, they adopted stressful city habits that led to their decline in health.

Compare the Hunzas to our culture. Experience tells me that our stressful lifestyles, poor dietary habits, and cultural expectations make it difficult for younger generations to live as long as the Hunzas. I've even had patients say, "If this is what old age is like, I don't want to be around that long."

In our culture, it seems as though we are dead at fifty and buried by sixty-five. After all, for many, fifty is the age when chronic illness hits; sixty-five is the age when we've reached the end of our productive years (i.e., retirement age). Age is something to be feared, not respected.

Unfortunately, many who wish to retire by sixty-five can't enjoy it because of health issues or the lack of retirement funds.

The Bible references the longevity of humankind and the awesome responsibility we have as stewards of what we've been given:

- All of our days are determined by God; he has appointed his limits that man cannot exceed. Job 14:5
- We are appointed stewards of what God has given us. 1 Corinthians 4:1
- To whom much is given, much is required. Luke 12:48

Caring for our bodies is certainly a tall order. We've been given one vessel in which to live our existence on this earth. It's up to us to make it count, no matter how many years are given.

> **The body is in a continuous state of fluctuation and adaptation to its environment.**
>
> —Virgil Strang, DC

Early in my career, I learned an important concept called the *biological continuum.* It states that a person's health is in a continual state of fluctuation throughout his or her lifetime, as represented by the diagram in Figure 1. below:

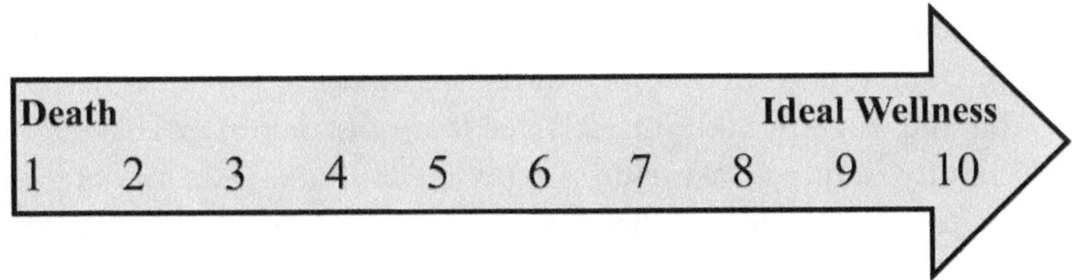

Each day when we climb out of bed, we look in the mirror and see the same image. We look the same and feel the same, so the belief that is reinforced is, we must be the same. You are the same person but your body chemistry can change from day to day, based on the things you did the day before. You're sowing seeds with the things you eat and drink and with the thoughts you think. The biological continuum tells of the potential for gaining health if you've lost it and maintaining health if you have it. Again, health doesn't happen by chance. Begin sowing the right seeds now!

A multitude of factors influence a person's health throughout his or her lifetime, such as diet, stress, toxins, rest, and the air we breathe. And now beliefs are added to the list.

I believe God didn't create you to be sick. Everyone should expect to be a ten on the biological continuum. Unfortunately, that expectation and reality are moving farther apart for many Americans. Life expectancy has slowly increased but at the expense of suffering from more chronic illnesses. I don't believe this is a fair exchange.

Where do you fit on the biological continuum? Hopefully you're a ten, but wherever you are on the scale, I hope your goal is to become a ten or to stay a ten.

> **The power that made the body heals the body. It happens no other way.**
>
> —B. J. Palmer
> son of D. D. Palmer
> founder of the chiropractic profession

What are your beliefs? Do you believe the power that made your body also heals your body? Or do you believe that the power to heal comes from your doctor or medications? Whatever you believe, to a certain extent you're right. Your beliefs determine your reality. Your beliefs have a powerful influence on your health. I encourage everyone to read *The Biology of Belief: Unleashing the Power of Consciousness, Matter & Miracles* by Bruce Lipton, PhD. It will open your eyes to how environment and beliefs influence your life and health.

Your life will flow in the direction of your most dominant beliefs. One of the healthiest things we can do is to periodically take inventory of those belief systems and evaluate if they are serving us in a positive way. Likewise, one of the most limiting things we can do is to hold onto outdated beliefs that keep us from moving forward.

One of the false beliefs I commonly hear is that your health is limited by your genes. A more accurate belief would be: faulty genetics don't hold you hostage. Your *environment* activates or inhibits your genes. An entire scientific field called epigenetics has come about from our understanding of the influence of environment on genetic expression. Epigenetics has proven that genes are response mechanisms that are activated or inhibited by your environment. Our genes continuously react the same way because we never change our environment.

What creates our environment? Quite often errors in diet and a high-stress level are the primary factors that negatively influence genetics. Stress chemicals suppress the immune system and alter gene expression. If you don't like the result, you must change your environment to get a better result.

Even in cases where genetics cause health issues, there's still hope. In chapter 9, I discuss a common genetic defect called the MTHFR SNiP (selective nucleotide polymorphism) that's common among many Americans. Statistics say you may have this defect and not even know it, as it's estimated to affect 60-80 percent of the population. The effects of this genetic defect can be countered through targeted nutrition. In fact, most people who have this defect but don't know they have it are being treated for its effects, such as diabetes or heart disease. So even if conventional medicine has no recognized therapy for the defect, there's still hope.

Remember, perfect health is more than just feeling good. Dorland's medical dictionary defines health as "a state of optimal physical, mental, and social well-being and not just the absence of disease or infirmity." It's a triune. Physical health is incomplete without the other two.

The reason the idea that "I am healthy if I feel good" is so deceiving is because it creates a false sense of reality and reinforces the notion that we'll deal with our health if we feel bad. This notion has permeated our society in so many ways. I hear it all the time when I talk to people. They think they are healthy simply because they feel okay when they aren't. High blood pressure and diabetes are two examples. Often a heart attack is the first symptom of high blood pressure. I've seen patients who had no warning signs before the big one, only to find out they had significant blockage of the coronary arteries.

Also diabetes is running rampant in our society, yet many people don't know they have blood sugar problems until critical damage has been done to their bodies.

The same applies to many forms of cancer. Many years ago I remember reading about the mechanisms that cause cancer in *Robbins Pathologic Basis of Disease*. What struck me was the reminder that cancer can exist in the body for seven to fifteen years before it is detectable by any means of diagnosis; further evidence that the most accurate technology has its limitations.

The story below is a real life example of this point.

Distance runner Jim Fixx became famous as a marathon runner in the early 1980s. In fact, he authored several books on the subject of healthy living through running.

Fixx was only fifty-two when he died of a massive heart attack. He was found lying on the side of a Vermont highway after collapsing while out for his daily run. An autopsy later revealed that Fixx had nearly 100 percent blockage of his coronary arteries. I'm sure if someone had asked Fixx how healthy he was prior to his death, however, he would have emphatically said, "I'm a ten."

If you're like me, the first question that comes to my mind is how could a man so physically fit have 100 percent blockage of his coronary arteries? On the surface it doesn't make sense. At the time, the cause of his artery disease was attributed to a genetic predisposition since his parents also reportedly suffered from heart disease. It was also reported that he had a history of unhealthy living in his younger years, which certainly could have shortened his lifespan. Could it be that his running accelerated his artery disease and shortened his lifespan to an even greater degree? Today's research would suggest that could indeed be the case.

In 1984, the year Jim Fixx died, medical research did not understand the effects of free radicals and advanced aging. Now the concept of tissue damage from free radicals has been well documented. In fact, medical professionals such as Dr. Kenneth Cooper and Dr. Russell Blaylock have written entire books on the subject.

Fixx participated in a sport that produces large amounts of destructive free radicals inside the body. Even though running has long been associated with good health, it is safe to say he was loading himself up with free radicals every time he ran. The constant bombardment of free radicals over the course of his life had to be a contributing factor to his shortened lifespan. How do I know this? Read the section on free radicals and exercise in chapter 4. It will support why I can make such a bold statement.

The body can only take so much of the free-radical assault before it breaks down—even in a healthy athlete like Jim Fixx.

In the next chapter I'll take a look at where we stand in health care compared to the rest of the world. This gives a compelling case for change if there ever was one.

CHAPTER 2

An Objective Comparison of the United States to Other Nations

Technology is wonderful, but it has its limitations. In the United States we have imaging technology that can see inside the body and even give us computer images of how the body is functioning. I'm thankful we have such wonderful technology, but simple wisdom tells us technology cannot replace the fundamentals that keep us healthy. Technology does not prioritize our food choices or exercise. Both are core aspects of prevention. Even with our advancements in technology, a quick look at current statistical data on the health of our population suggests that a large percentage of our population is suffering. I believe this is a strong indication that the health of our nation is declining.

Even with all the advancements in technology, chronic pain has risen to nearly epidemic proportions in our country. Current estimates indicate that nearly 100 million Americans live with chronic pain. (That's one-third of the population.[1]) It is estimated that employee lost time from chronic pain and poor health are costing US employers $576 billion annually.[2]

As chronic pain rises, more people are turning to over-the-counter (OTC) pain relievers (aspirin, acetaminophen, and ibuprofen) under the impression that these drugs are safe because they are sold without a prescription. People are self-medicating with ever-increasing frequency and research is revealing the repercussions of this trend.

Studies have identified long-term (five years or more) daily use of aspirin as a significant risk factor for developing breast cancer. One study stated the risk of developing breast cancer increased by an average of 81 percent with long-term use.[3] The same study stated long-term daily use of ibuprofen increases the risk of developing breast cancer by 51 percent.

Other studies have shown similar findings related to aspirin use.[4] Taking more than fourteen aspirin per week increases your risk of pancreatic cancer by 86 percent.[5]

Long-term use of acetaminophen has been linked to hypertension and renal failure. Acetaminophen is now considered the number one cause of liver failure in the United States. The drug was documented as the primary cause of 42 percent of acute liver failures from 1998 to 2003. [6,7]

According to the *New England Journal of Medicine*, there is a lifetime maximum dosage for all OTC pain relievers. When these drugs are combined, it enhances the risk of organ failure. For acetaminophen the maximum lifetime dosage is one thousand tablets. Even consuming one a day for a year will double the risk of kidney failure within twenty years. Exceed five thousand tablets and it will increase your chances of organ failure by 800 percent.[8]

Acetaminophen is also known to deplete glutathione from the body. Glutathione is a powerful antioxidant that protects the cells from damage and also serves as a major detoxifier of drugs and toxic chemicals. Glutathione depletion can cause serious problems. Wait, there's more:

OTC pain relievers are the leading cause of dialysis every year. They are the leading cause of liver damage in children (thirty-two thousand cases per year). They cause seventeen thousand deaths each year from gastrointestinal (GI) bleeding. This has been comparable to the number of deaths from AIDS historically.

Granted, some of these statistics are purely from people overdosing on pain medications. But how many are from people who are using the proper dosages but over extended periods of time, unaware of the danger that lurks ahead? When I see statistics like this, it makes me ask, "What is going on? Why are so many people suffering from chronic pain when we have all the technology to address these issues?" The simple answer is, technology, whether in the form of medications or advanced imaging methods, are not effectively addressing chronic pain in our culture. Some medications are even creating larger issues, especially relating to severe side effects.

OTC pain medications have warning labels on the bottles that "inform" people about the possible repercussions, but people are rolling the dice and taking their chances.

It is apparent from these studies that self-medicating has become a real problem. I think the major factor in creating chronic pain syndromes is the busy, stressful lifestyles people lead. People push themselves beyond their limits, and it takes a toll on the body in many ways. Self-medicating appears to be an attempt by consumers to cope with chronic pain.

I think this would also call into question the wisdom of making higher potency pain relievers available without a prescription. I know many of these medications were released to the OTC market to reduce the need for doctor visits, thereby reducing medical costs. But the trend of self-medicating among the population is not showing promising results.

At the same time, there are natural methods that help immensely with chronic pain that do not have negative side effects. In my clinical experience, chiropractic adjustments, acupuncture, massage therapy, and natural anti-inflammatories such as resveratrol, turmeric and curcumin are very effective at restoring structural balance and addressing chronic pain at its source. Even better, they have no side effects if utilized properly. These are included in what the government calls "alternative medicine." For thousands upon thousands of people, they are not alternative at all. Chiropractic is a way of life for many, including my family and me. These natural healing methods are grossly underutilized thanks in part to limited third-party reimbursement and a limited public perception of their benefits.

Since chiropractic is an approach that is unknown to many people, it often takes a thorough explanation of how it is different from a conventional approach and why the chiropractic approach is necessary to get patients to commit to care plans and not just patch things up. Most chiropractors do a very good job of spending the time necessary to provide educational training.

Based on the previous statistics, higher utilization of chiropractic care would save lives and reduce costs associated with organ dialysis and organ transplants (as well as prevent needless suffering). Unfortunately the patients with the highest chronicity like arthritis and degenerative diseases, especially in the elderly, are given the least amount of financial support from third-party payers. This is quite frustrating to say the least.

Now please indulge me for a moment as I continue to look closely at where we are as a nation in terms of world health.

The United States is 5 percent of the world's population but consumes 70 percent of the world's medications. Think about that. This statistic reflects the overdependence of our society on medications and the desire for a "quick fix." Unfortunately the quick fix seldom addresses the true cause of the problem.

According to World Health Organization statistics, the United States ranks thirty-fourth in life expectancy and has the fifth highest infant mortality rate of all industrialized nations. Infant mortality rate refers to the survival of an infant through the first five years of life (tables 1 and 1A below).

Table 1: Life Expectancy (World Health Organization, 2015)

Overall Rank	Country	Overall Life Expectancy	Male Rank	Male Life Expectancy	Female Rank	Female Life Expectancy
1	Japan	84	5	80	1	87
2	Switzerland	83	2	81	5	85
2	Spain	83	5	80	2	86
2	Singapore	83	2	81	5	85
2	San Marino	83	1	83	11	84
2	Italy	83	5	80	5	85
2	Australia	83	5	80	5	85
2	Andorra	83	16	79	2	86
9	Sweden	82	5	80	11	84
9	Norway	82	5	80	11	84
9	New Zealand	82	5	80	11	84
9	Monaco	82	16	79	5	85
9	Luxembourg	82	5	80	11	84
9	Israel	82	2	81	11	84
9	Iceland	82	2	81	11	84
9	France	82	16	79	5	85
9	Cyprus	82	5	80	11	84
9	Canada	82	5	80	11	84
19	United Kingdom	81	16	79	22	83
19	Republic of Korea	81	24	78	5	85
19	Portugal	81	24	78	11	84
19	Netherlands	81	16	79	22	83
19	Malta	81	16	79	34	82
19	Ireland	81	16	79	22	83
19	Greece	81	16	79	11	84

Overall Rank	Country	Overall Life Expectancy	Male Rank	Male Life Expectancy	Female Rank	Female Life Expectancy
19	Germany	81	16	79	22	83
19	Finland	81	24	78	11	84
19	Austria	81	16	79	11	84
29	Slovenia	80	33	77	22	83
29	Lebanon	80	24	78	34	82
29	Denmark	80	24	78	34	82
29	Chile	80	33	77	22	83
29	Belgium	80	24	78	22	83
34	United States	79	37	76	36	81
34	Qatar	79	16	79	45	80
34	Nauru	79	45	75	22	83
34	Cuba	79	37	76	36	81
34	Costa Rica	79	33	77	36	81
34	Colombia	79	37	76	22	83
40	Kuwait	78	24	78	53	79
40	Czech Republic	78	45	75	36	81
40	Croatia	78	51	74	36	81
40	Barbados	78	45	75	36	81

Table 1A: Under-Five Mortality Rate per 1,000 Live Births (World Health Organization, 2015)

Rank	Country	Under-Five Mortality Rate
1	Turkey	13.5
2	Mexico	13.2
3	Chile	8.1
4	Slovakia	7.3
5	United States	6.5
6	Hungary	5.9
7	New Zealand	5.7
8	Poland	5.2
9	Canada	4.9

Rank	Country	Under-Five Mortality Rate
10	Greece	4.6
11	France	4.3
12	United Kingdom	4.2
13	Spain	4.1
13	Belgium	4.1
15	Israel	4.0
16	Switzerland	3.9
17	Australia	3.8
17	Netherlands	3.8
19	Germany	3.7
20	Portugal	3.6
20	Ireland	3.6
22	Italy	3.5
22	Denmark	3.5
24	Austria	3.5
24	Czech Republic	3.4
24	South Korea	3.4
27	Sweden	3.0
28	Estonia	2.9
29	Japan	2.7
30	Slovenia	2.6
30	Norway	2.6
32	Finland	2.3
33	Iceland	2.0
34	Luxembourg	1.9

At the time this book went to press, early estimates for life expectancy in 2017 suggest the United States has slipped even further to fifty-third, according to data website geoba.se.[9] Clearly the numbers are not heading in the right direction.

When you compare life expectancy to health-care spending, the picture becomes even cloudier. Table 2 shows how the United States compared to other nations in health-care spending for 2010. Fast-forward to 2015, Congressional Budget Office statistics show the United States funded 20.6 percent of its entire GDP on health care, at an average annual cost of more than $8,500 per person. This represents a $3 billion increase in just five years.[10]

Table 2: Health-Care Spending For 2010

2010 Health Spending as Percent of GDP

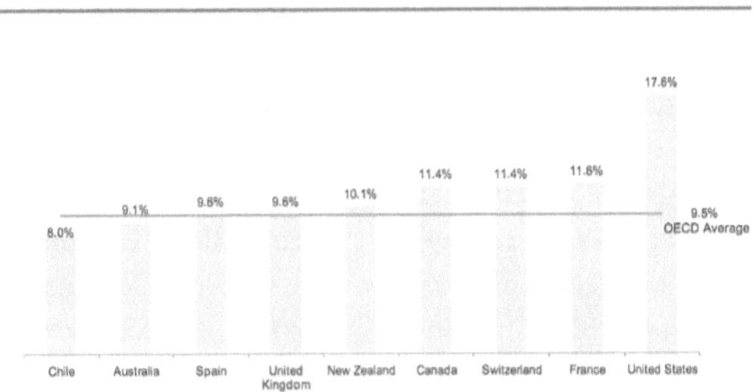

Clearly we cannot sustain that level of spending. In the financial world they talk about ROI, return on investment. What are we getting for our healthcare dollars? That's where it gets even more confusing.

The only category in which the United States leads is in health-care spending and by a wide margin. Populations in other countries are not only living longer but they also are doing so at a lower cost. Few countries ranked ahead of us have all the technological advances that we have in the United States. If technology were the sole answer to our health-care problems, we would have solved the healthcare puzzle by now and other countries would be learning from us.

I submit to you that what we are looking at is really not health care that helps people in these other nations live longer. It has more to do with their culture and lifestyles. Many nations have food supplies that are naturally grown, with less emphasis on synthetic chemicals and preservatives; in fact some chemicals used in our food supply have been banned in Europe for years. In some countries, their lifestyles operate at a much slower pace with much lower stress levels.

For the Hunzas, there is no crime or stress. The staple of their diet is fresh fruits and vegetables. In case you were wondering (as I was) why the Hunzas were not listed on the life expectancy chart, it's probably because they are a reclusive tribal people mostly unknown to the outside world.

Citizens of Norway (tied for ninth on the life expectancy list) regularly consume a high-fat diet, yet they have extremely low rates of heart disease. Citizens of Japan consume a high-carbohydrate diet by our standards. They also have a longer life expectancy. Even European nations like France and the United Kingdom, which have similar diets to ours, fare better than the United States. Their portion sizes are much smaller, so the health impact is much less than the supersized portion sizes found in our country.

A patient of mine who was born and raised in France once told me how much of a culture shock it was adjusting to the large portion sizes when he moved to the United States. For instance, a large soft drink in France is 12 ounces. A large soft drink here is twice that amount, and you have the option to supersize it, taking the quantity all the way up to 32 ounces. One 12-ounce soda contains the sugar equivalent of four candy bars. You do the math on the 32-ounce soda. Diet sodas are even worse because of artificial sweeteners. Keep this in mind as you read chapter 6, "The Diabetes Epidemic."

Clearly differences in culture and cultural habits have to contribute to greater longevity and better health.

Positive Consumer Trends: Higher Demand for Vitamins and Natural Products

In the United States, consumer spending for items like vitamins and natural foods has risen at an exponential rate, suggesting there is a shift occurring as people are searching for new methods to stay healthy. In fact, it is estimated that wellness products are now a $500 billion industry. This is an increase of $200 billion in just five years. It is estimated wellness products will become a trillion-dollar industry by 2020.[11] This is a positive trend that needs to continue, but with a word of caution: as much as this data suggests that people are seeking alternatives to taking large amounts of prescription medication, it's important for consumers to understand the difference between natural and synthetic vitamins, ensuring they are taking the right supplements for improving their health. (This will be covered in chapter 9). I commonly see people taking the wrong type of vitamins, unaware that certain types of vitamins provide little health benefit. The good news is, I know consumers just need some direction on how to make better choices. The bad news is, it seems they are not getting it from healthcare providers on a broad scale. That's why consumers are taking matters into their own hands and bypassing the professionals.

I believe we are rapidly moving away from the age of placing all the responsibility for one's health onto doctors. This means the role of physicians is changing from being the expert and the healer to that of being a coach and a mentor who provides guidance so consumers can make wiser choices. Will health care providers embrace this change? Only time will tell.

There are challenges to this gradual shift:

Challenge #1: Unfortunately, as our regulatory agencies see a growing trend in consumers' use of supplements, tighter regulations are making it much more difficult for supplement companies to produce and market their products effectively, often under the disguise of "consumer safety." In the end, this makes it even more difficult for consumers because products that can be beneficial are slowly being removed from the market or, at the very least, are more tightly regulated.

Challenge #2: With a rapidly growing body of research that is increasingly technical, the information is evolving so rapidly that physicians are challenged with communicating valid health information to consumers to help them in their decision-making. Physicians of all disciplines must find creative ways to bridge the gap between research data and public knowledge.

The Statistic You Do Not Want to Be

On a positive note, statistics show we are living longer than we were even ten years ago. As life expectancy rises, however, chronic illness has also steadily increased. If you look at disease rates over time, cancer and heart disease were relatively unheard of in the early 1900s. Some would say this is a result of shorter life expectancies. I don't think so. I think we're seeing the long-term effects of the slow but progressive degradation of our food supply, along with an exponential increase in the toxic exposure that is causing the rise in chronic disease rates. In fact, the data suggests that chronic degenerative diseases are consuming our culture and rapidly draining our financial resources. Even our medical system says we are losing the battle with this monster called chronic illness.

I encourage you to read the article cited for this statistic; it was published in the *Journal of the American Medical Association,* August 14, 2013. "The State of US Health 1990–2010: The Burden of Diseases, Injuries, and Risk Factors"[12] paints a disturbing picture of where we are and where we are heading. The clear message in this article is that we cannot sustain the pace we're on in terms of our approach to chronic illness and the cost associated with that approach. This should sound an alarm with *everyone* that a change in direction is overdue. Will the authorities continue to do the same things over and over, expecting a different result? Will consumers be open to change? Time will tell.

But where is the money going and why is it so expensive to provide health care? Looking deeper, here's what the data shows: take a look at the leading causes of death in the United States. That's your first clue. Keep in mind, this is deaths per year, according to the Centers for Disease Control, 2013:

1. Heart disease: 611,105
2. Cancer: 584,881
3. Lung disease: 149,205
4. Accidents (unintentional injuries, including deaths from routine medical care): 130,557
5. Stroke (cerebrovascular diseases): 128,978
6. Alzheimer's disease: 84,767
7. Diabetes: 75,578
8. Influenza and pneumonia: 56,979
9. Kidney disease: 47,112
10. Intentional self-harm (suicide): 41,149

You may notice the majority of my focus in this book is on these ten diseases, especially heart disease. Why?

- These are the core illnesses for which we have not found an answer.
- The combination of all of them together is rapidly becoming an insurmountable burden to our society.

Understanding the origin of heart disease gives us tremendous insight into the origins of other diseases. They all have a similar underlying etiology at the cellular and molecular level. Hopefully that will become clear in the pages that follow. It's hard to fix something when you're not focused on the source of the problem.

Overall, the leading causes of death have stayed largely the same over the last thirty years in spite of years of research and new advancements in treating them. In fact, death from heart disease increased in 2016 for the first time in decades. When you understand the bigger picture, it becomes apparent that these diseases are somewhat self-induced. There is a unique and intense anguish that I have seen in patients who ultimately realize it was their lifestyle choices that created the diseases with which they are diagnosed. It's an anguish I would not wish on anyone. I've had patients with chronic illnesses attend my lectures and say to me afterwards, "I've been a lifelong smoker." "I never learned how to eat a healthy diet." "Did I do this to myself?" Quite often the answer is yes. The look in their eyes motivates me to keep explaining, keep educating. That's why I say to them, start making changes now, before it's too late.

In the end, if our lifestyles have brought on these diseases, we have the power to fix them with early intervention and lifestyle changes. The body is very resilient; it responds to healthy changes but they must be consistent to get lasting results.

Our resources are draining rapidly, and time is of the essence to find cost-effective answers. This is not about a quick trip to the emergency room to get stitches for a cut or a trip to the doctor to treat a cold. It's the chronic nature that makes these diseases so threatening. In reality, all of these diseases have a common ground that is not being effectively addressed with our advanced medical technology. Hopefully this will become clear as you read the remaining chapters.

The true cost associated with these illnesses is multifaceted with the development of new drugs and the cost of long-term care rising each year. A large portion of medical research is conducted to find ways to treat the illnesses and, to a lesser extent, find ways to prevent them. The "treating illness" part is what gets the vast majority of attention and research dollars. These statistics support what I am saying:

According to the National Cancer Institute, funding for cancer research alone has reached a whopping $5.2 billion per year.[13]

And the *Journal of the American Medical Association* reports that total funding for all medical research has exceeded $110 billion per year.[14]

These figures don't include the cost of long-term care for debilitating conditions. The key point is that long-term care is provided *after* the conditions have become debilitating. This is significant because it reflects that the preventive measures we have in our medical system are not stopping the progression of these diseases. They are prolonging life, but the progression of the illnesses is escalating. In fact that is the trend for all of these diseases, not just one of them. People are living longer with the disease, which adds to the overall cost of caring for them. The previous article on the state of US healthcare even suggests that they are pleased that they are prolonging lives, even though more and more people are developing chronic illness. I think we can do better if we make some cultural changes.

My goodness, are we all just sitting ducks waiting to be diagnosed with a debilitating illness? I can say with confidence it doesn't have to be that way if we take the right preventive measures far enough in advance to truly stop the onset and progression. This is where we as a society are falling short.

Even though prevention of disease gets much less attention and funding, we know a lot about how disease develops and how to prevent disease from occurring. Eventually the knowledge of health and disease progresses to a point where you have to apply what you've learned. My continuing education seminars frequently remind me of this vital truth. I regularly attend seminars that provide tremendous insight into the cause and prevention of various diseases we are battling. And it's all scientifically based information, taken directly from scientific literature. My colleague, Dr. Brandon Lundell, eloquently described the disease process as the body's internal reaction to toxic environmental conditions. Much of our internal environment comes from the things we eat or allow into our bodies. Then, the cells must have the correct nerve supply to function correctly. It's basic physiology. If we change the environment, the body's reaction will change accordingly. Healing of any condition requires improvement in the environmental conditions in the body.

It's a sad reality that we are seeing more evidence that new illnesses are being created or worsened by the proposed treatments for these diseases. Statin drugs, for example, are being dispensed not only to lower cholesterol levels but also to prevent heart attack and strokes (numbers one and five on the disease list). Yet we know from published studies that prolonged use of statin drugs has created an entirely new set of problems that will require long-term solutions. Diabetes (number seven on the list) and obesity are at epidemic levels, and statins are known to greatly increase the risk of developing diabetes, obesity, peripheral neuropathy, dementia, and cancer.[15,16] It's not just from prolonged use either. Two years on a statin drug increases the risk of painful diabetic neuropathy by an incredible 1,600 percent, suggesting the risk increases with longer use.[17]

And that's just the beginning of seeing the big picture of modern health care. Alzheimer's disease presents even bigger problems. What a horrible disease. Of all the chronic diseases we are facing today, Alzheimer's disease is the one that many experts have said will become an insurmountable financial burden to our health-care system by the year 2025—greater than heart disease, cancer, and the rest of the top diseases combined. According to a University of Southern California study, baby boomers will drive the explosion in Alzheimer's-related costs in the coming decades.[18]

It seems the common perception is that we have no insight into the cause of this dreaded disease. Yet, in multiple seminars I have attended over the past two years, information was presented that confirms we *do* know what causes Alzheimer's disease. Actually there is no singular cause, but looking at the big picture, it appears that inflammation in key regions of the brain plays a large role in the onset and progression. Other possible causes include immune system reactions created from vaccines early in life and overuse of OTC pain medications, which creates changes in the brain structure and reduction of the antioxidant glutathione. Mineral toxicity, especially copper, iron, and aluminum, has also been implicated. Where do these minerals come from? Municipal drinking water, synthetic vitamins, and in the case of aluminum, preservatives used in vaccines. I'll cover many of these in later chapters.

Number ten on the cause of death list is suicide. Statistics suggest a large percentage of suicides occur with people who are already taking antidepressants and psychotropic medications. Widespread use of antidepressants is now being linked with violent behavior and suicide. In his book *Prozac Backlash: Overcoming the Dangers of Prozac, Zoloft, Paxil, and Other Antidepressants with Safe, Effective Alternatives,* Dr. Joseph Glenmullen offers insight into this growing problem. He says, "… the high rate of violence and suicide is being strongly linked with widespread use of antidepressants and psychotropic medications. The rise in suicides and shootings in recent years coincides with the large amount of people being placed on antidepressants. Approximately 28 million people currently take Selective Serotonin Reuptake Inhibitors (SSRIs) for depression. SSRIs have a long list of side effects; suicidal and violent behaviors are two of them."[19]

The research suggests that inflammatory activity in the gut and the brain are responsible for the chemical changes associated with depression and a host of other disorders.[20] This is a major reason why probiotics and high-dose omega-3 therapy are so effective in depression and behavioral disorders. There are genetic SNiP's that hinder the utilization of fats in the brain which accelerate the depletion of key enzymes within the brain itself, resulting in chemical imbalances. The effects of the SNiP's are magnified by stress and poor diet.[21] Fish oil is very effective in depression because it addresses inflammation at its source. The effectiveness is much greater when coupled with other lifestyle changes. I'll cover dietary fats in more detail in chapters 4 and 5. For now, just know that addressing the cause of depression starts with preventive lifestyle changes, especially diet, exercise, stress management and ramping up the omega 3's.

What about conservative treatment for depression? Some practitioners avoid the dreaded topic of conservative management because they don't have the time and some don't feel comfortable with the topic. However, this is a critical component to helping patients with depression.

Speaking of conservative management, did you know chiropractic adjustments have been shown to have a calming effect on the body by inhibiting the sympathetic nervous system? I have seen many patients over the years reduce or discontinue their antidepressants with a multi-disciplinary approach to care, i.e. chiropractic care, diet and other lifestyle modifications and mental health professional supervision.

Please understand, I am not against medicine or a medical approach to combating chronic illnesses. After looking at the statistical data, I am suggesting that we need to continue researching, learning, and discovering new ways of preventing illness instead of waiting for disease to develop and treating it after the fact.

Fortunately, more and more scientific literature is addressing the need for prevention. Approaching illness through conservative means is becoming more widespread, even in the medical profession. Anyone who looks closely at health-care trends in America over the last century will notice there have been two opposing camps with opposite approaches to health care. The dividing line between these two approaches has been wide.

On one side, you have the holistic practitioners, such as chiropractors, naturopaths, acupuncturists, and some (traditional) osteopaths, who have approached health care from a drug-free perspective. Spinal adjustments, nutritional supplements, stress relief activities such as Yoga or exercise and meditation / prayer are some of the primary treatment methods that holistic practitioners use with much success. On the other side lies the traditional medical approach, utilizing primarily drugs and surgery. However, with the growing body of knowledge on natural healing methods, there are an ever-increasing number of doctors on the fringe of mainstream medicine who are bypassing the traditional medical model in favor of a more holistic practice. With increasing frequency, medical doctors are churning out books on wellness topics like nutrition, whole body detoxification, exercise, and other holistic topics. Right in front of our eyes we are seeing health care come full circle, from high-tech pharmaceuticals back to more natural approaches. Even more eye-opening, some doctors are turning away from the conventional medical practice and converting to a more conservative natural approach. This is a welcome change spawned by necessity. The question is, can we make the transition fast enough?

Why in the world would so many doctors broaden their approach, turning away from the traditional medical practice? Believe me, I've read scathing commentary from medical insiders who don't think very highly of the message these progressive doctors are sending. *Heresy* and *quackery* are some of the words being tossed out. I think these doctors clearly see the impending health crisis, and they know we cannot overcome the problems of the twenty-first century by using the same paradigm that brought us to this point.

Imagine trying to stop a speeding locomotive that is barreling out of control knowing you don't have the tools or the resources to stop it. Then you suddenly realize the solution was there in front of you all along. Sometimes it takes a new paradigm, a new approach to solve old problems. These progressive doctors are joining the ranks of chiropractors and other holistic doctors who have preached a conservative message for over a hundred years. To all of these doctors I say welcome home. Now let's work together to stop this speeding locomotive.

How Did We Get Here?

> "The doctor of the future will give no medicine but will interest his patients in the care of the human frame, in diet, and in the cause and prevention of disease."

> "Surgery, diet, antiseptics—these three are the vital things of the future in preserving the health of humanity. There

were never so many able, active minds at work on the problems of diseases as now, and all their discoveries are tending to the simple truth—that you can't improve on nature."

—Thomas Edison, 1902

The path that brought us to where we are is a little complicated to say the least. Actually it has its roots as far back as the 1800s with the modern evolution of the germ theory. Infectious diseases were commonplace in those days. As new discoveries were being made in the study of microbiology (germs) and its effects on the body, medicine adopted a pharmaceutical approach to combating those microbes. The pharmaceutical industry quickly became a multimillion, multibillion and now a multitrillion-dollar industry by the mid-twentieth century. The power to heal was placed in the medication of the day.

The landscape of disease has changed from those early days. Especially in the United States, we no longer live with the constant threat of infectious epidemics and plagues. Even the once dreaded HIV virus, known as the cause of Acquired Immune Deficiency Syndrome (AIDS), is now seventy fourth on the list of death from illness. Instead, chronic illnesses like heart disease, stroke, cancer, and Alzheimer's disease have moved up the list of illnesses that threaten humankind. Health-care technology has changed rapidly to address these issues, mostly through advances in pharmaceutical technology.

Problem: as pharmaceuticals have become more sophisticated, an ever-growing list of side effects has emerged. Reality: side effects occur because the medications are interrupting other vital physiological processes.

As we understand more about the cause of heart disease, cancer, and all the other chronic diseases, we are learning they are lifestyle-induced illnesses. We know that poor dietary habits are a major factor in all chronic diseases. Logic would tell you that correcting these lifestyle factors should be a central part of fixing the problem. I can say with confidence, as a society we're not even close to where we need to be on preventive lifestyle changes. It's changing but we still have a long way to go.

With the ongoing rise in technology, the power and influence of "big pharma" on our health-care system has continued to grow and grow and grow. Authors Ray Moynihan and Alan Cassels provide an excellent summary of this growth and influence in their 2006 book, *Selling Sickness:*

How the World's Largest Pharmaceutical Companies Are Turning Us All into Patients. I have included a short summary of this book as a point of emphasis and to show the powerful influence pharmaceutical companies have on our healthcare system and our research dollars.

"This book reveals how widening the boundaries of illness and lowering the threshold for treatments is creating millions of new patients and billions in new profits, in turn threatening to bankrupt health-care systems all over the world."

Not a good recipe for cost reduction in an era of high cost medicine.

There are many factors involved in the direction we are heading in health care. The locomotive of big pharma drives the direction of our research clear down to the methods used to treat diseases of our day. Any change in direction, or even slight modifications in direction, goes against the grain of the accepted norm. Even if physicians believe in alternative health care, it's difficult to survive when labeled as a heretic. The question I continually ask myself is can we improve the health of our country by addressing more of the lifestyle factors that cause these modern diseases? I think the answer is an emphatic yes. It's really not that complicated. By creating a new model of healthcare, indirectly we make the old model obsolete. The new model is preventative, which integrates the best of medicine and the best of conservative management to form a better system. Keep reading.

The Short Summary

We have an aging population, primarily the baby boomers, who are suffering from chronic illnesses in ever-increasing numbers. Our research dollars are directed toward helping those who already have cancer, diabetes, and heart disease. We have two younger generations that are developing the same diseases as baby boomers at nearly half the age. This is the core piece of the financial burden. Who provides for the younger generations as they are afflicted with these diseases? Based on statistics alone, the preventive measures we are using are not slowing down the progression of chronic diseases, and the diseases are affecting younger generations. Lifestyle factors are a major player in the disease process for all three generations. Modifying our approach to these diseases is appropriate and necessary, but we are stuck in a narrow paradigm that has a high cost. This just about sums it up. But what are we missing? It's prevention, and the research supports that conclusion.

What Prevention Addresses

Prevention addresses the core issues that cause illnesses to occur in the first place. Any discussion of prevention has to include vitamin deficiencies. For example, take a look at some of the research on the preventive aspects of vitamin D.

Despite all the efforts to immunize for the flu every year, look at this data that was published in medical journals from 2006 to 2010. This literature suggests that the primary trigger for seasonal cases of influenza and pneumonia is related to clinically low vitamin D levels. In other words, vitamin D makes the call to send the cavalry to clean up the foreign invaders. Low vitamin D intake causes lowered resistance to infection.[22,23,24]

Researchers have determined that vitamin D increases blood levels of a peptide (a single protein) called LL-37. LL-37 improves the immune response to a wide variety of infections, thereby increasing resistance. The bugs don't wake up one day and decide to get nasty. The host (you) becomes susceptible to the bugs from lowered resistance. What a novel idea that we have the power to fight off these microbes if we have the right ammunition.

These articles point out that exposure to sunlight is the best producer of vitamin D. Even though this sounds easy in theory, it's not as easy as it sounds. Getting the maximum dosage of vitamin D from sunlight requires at least ¾ of the body to be exposed to the sun for a minimum of 45 minutes, 3-4 times a week. In other words, limited exposure from having your arm hanging out the car window or from the sun shining through the glass on your face is not enough. Vitamin D deficiency has become even more prevalent because of reduced sun exposure brought about from the rapid increase in skin related cancers. Therefore, vitamin D supplementation is *required* in areas where sun exposure is restricted, which is a good portion of the country, especially in the winter months. It should be no coincidence that flu season typically occurs in the fall and winter months when a large percentage of the population is indoors without sunlight for months at a time. If you spend a lot of time outdoors with ample skin exposure, chances are you will not require vitamin D supplementation.

Here's an interesting fact: cases of influenza have *not* declined in spite of a mass increase in flu vaccinations. And it is estimated that those with vitamin D deficiency experience 39 percent higher health-care costs than those with normal vitamin D levels.[25] Maybe the impact of flu season will be reduced when we start monitoring vitamin D levels in susceptible individuals, which is just about everyone.

Even though the articles don't mention this directly, many people become more sedentary in the winter months. And, especially through the holidays, overconsumption of sugary foods increases, which also lowers resistance.

Many articles I have read say that clinically low vitamin D levels are common throughout the population. This means that even in our modern society, we still have vitamin deficiencies. We also have "authorities" who insist that vitamin deficiencies are a thing of the past. I'm not sure where they obtain their information, but these authorities are quite mistaken. As you read on, you will understand the reasons for vitamin deficiencies more clearly.

There is also promising research on vitamin D and cancer prevention. This research indicates that many forms of cancer are driven by an inappropriate immune response. One study emphasized that approximately three-fourths of the population is grossly deficient in vitamin D. Researchers have stated that low vitamin D is a causal mechanism for cancer of the breast and colon. They conclude that most of these cancers could be prevented with adequate vitamin D levels in the blood.

Another study that appeared in the journal *Neurology* has suggested a link between low vitamin D intake and multiple sclerosis.[26]

Still other studies have linked vitamin D levels to autism and behavioral disorders.[27] Widespread chronic pain has also been linked to low vitamin D levels.[28,29]

I would recommend having your vitamin D level tested. It's a simple blood test with a nominal cost. Doctors Data (www.doctorsdata.com) is one of many labs with a simple blood spot test for vitamin D. If it strengthens your resistance and effectively prevents the flu, chronic pain, and even cancer, it would be well worth the cost. Monitoring blood levels is the best way to assure you are not overdosing.

This is just one of many vitamin deficiencies that are common in our society. Many disorders cause malabsorption of nutrients. Poor dietary habits lead to a condition called leaky gut syndrome, in which the lining of the gut is damaged, allowing foreign matter to enter the blood stream. Leaky gut syndrome can lead to harmful bacterial overgrowth in the intestines, eventually causing autoimmune disorders as the immune system begins to attack the body's own tissue.

We commonly hear about the importance of calcium intake to maintain strong bones. Some authors are now saying that Vitamin D, magnesium, and vitamin K are perhaps more important than calcium intake for strong bones and a healthy body. Harvard University school of medicine professor Dr. Walter Willett says one rarely needs calcium supplementation with adequate levels of Vitamin D. He even suggests that calcium supplementation in high amounts can be hazardous to your health. Others have suggested that a high level of calcium opens the channels in the brain that initiate pain in the body (the pain gate).

The ratio of calcium to magnesium in the blood is very important for health and wellbeing. Carolyn Dean, M.D. says the optimum ratio of calcium to magnesium in the blood is 1:1; yet the average American measures about 10:1. This suggests most Americans are over consuming calcium and grossly under consuming magnesium. Vitamin D depends on adequate magnesium for proper absorption and utilization. Magnesium also plays a role in bone health, brain health, and in decreasing inflammatory reactions in the body. Magnesium also blocks the pain producing nerves that cause fibromyalgia, an agonizing nerve condition. In addition, Magnesium plays a role in nearly 800 vital enzyme reactions in the body. Magnesium deficiency is also linked with hypertension and high blood pressure.

The source of the magnesium is an important factor in the absorption of vitamin D. The best source of magnesium for proper absorption is magnesium malate, glycinate, or citrate. The combination of magnesium and malic acid in particular aids in energy production in the cells while serving the protective role described above.

Be Careful! Using the wrong type of minerals can be just as harmful as not using any minerals at all. Magnesium oxide is a common form of magnesium used in commercial vitamin supplements that is difficult to absorb and can cause kidney stones in certain individuals.

Another very common nutrient deficiency is vitamin K. This misunderstood vitamin is often deficient because of an overall lack of green leafy vegetables in the American diet. Many people with blood clotting issues are advised to limit intake of green leafy vegetables due to the role of vitamin K1 in blood clotting. There are actually four different forms of vitamin K that serve different roles in the body: K1, K2, K4 and K7. Vitamin K2, 4 and 7 are involved in helping the body absorb and utilize vitamin D and calcium. Deficiencies will limit the absorption and utilization of Vitamin D and cause calcium to collect in the arteries.

Always seek the guidance of a qualified professional when taking supplements that are unfamiliar to you, at least until you can acquire enough knowledge to self-administer your own supplements.

This is just a short list of common nutrient deficiencies in our society today. As we acquire more knowledge on the effects of these deficiencies on the body, we will need to re-learn some things about nutrition to effectively address these issues.

When I reviewed the more recent data on vitamin D, magnesium and vitamin K, it became clear that it contradicts many of the current and accepted medical guidelines for these nutrients. Our bodies need more of these nutrients than we originally thought. They serve protective roles that were not discovered until recently. This is yet another example where medical professionals will need to discard old information as new information evolves. Prevention of problems associated with these deficiencies must start by addressing the lifestyle problems that created them.

Keep reading to learn more about the cause and prevention of modern diseases.

CHAPTER 3

The Disconnect between Science, the Public, and the Food Industry

> How many people would do things differently if they only knew the seeds they were sowing were going to manifest in disease later in life?
>
> —James Darnell DC

Recommendations for a low-fat diet along with an increase in grains and refined carbohydrates have their roots as far back as the early1900's, when the incidence of heart disease and stroke was quite low. Progressing through the 1940s, the incidence of heart disease and stroke gradually began to escalate. Could it be that it took twenty to thirty years for the effects of regular consumption of grains and refined foods to appear? Looking back, that certainly appears to be the case.

Low-fat diets really came to the forefront in the 1950s as fast-food restaurants became commonplace. Perhaps you have seen the old black-and-white photos of people sitting in their cars at the drive-in, chowing down on burgers, fries, and milk shakes.

At that time medical science was only beginning to understand the long-term effect of grains, carbohydrates, and refined oils on the body. It was slowly becoming evident that more and more people were developing cholesterol deposits in their arteries and these deposits were causing heart attacks and strokes. This forced medical science to investigate why so many cases of cholesterol deposits in the arteries and heart disease were suddenly appearing.[1] The logical conclusion was if people are dying from cholesterol deposits in their arteries, consuming too much cholesterol is the culprit, and therefore, limiting cholesterol is the solution.

They were right about some things but wrong about others. The part that was left out was a huge piece of the puzzle: since fat and cholesterol were labeled as the evil that was causing heart disease, all fat was labeled as bad. This led to even bigger problems because the body needs a certain amount of dietary fat and cholesterol to stay healthy. Low cholesterol levels never did and never will prevent heart disease. And, excessively low cholesterol can create problems for the body, as you will see in coming chapters.

The major piece that was missing in the low-fat craze was "not all fats are created equal." Some fats are actually good for the body and are necessary for good health. But the fear of fat had begun among our medical professionals and our citizens, and it quickly snowballed into a movement.

Fast-forward from the 1950s through the 1970s, and the recommendations for a low-fat diet transitioned to include even higher quantities of grains and carbohydrates, along with a steady increase in the consumption of refined oils. Margarine came to the forefront in American homes because of the low-fat recommendations of the 1950s.

I started practice in 1993, and even at that time I saw evidence suggesting that low-fat diets were causing problems, but it was not clear yet exactly what was missing. Now we know and the picture is not pretty.

Progressing through the late 1990s, the evidence continued to show that there was more to the story of heart disease than just dietary fat intake. We now know the primary culprit that ramps up cholesterol in the blood and clogs the arteries is refined, processed food. Processed carbs are converted to cholesterol. Processed carbs stress the sugar handling capability of the body, especially the liver and the pancreas, sparking a chain reaction within the body. The statistics tell the story because the 1950s was the decade when the real transition to processed food began, and the 1970s cemented the deal. The rise in heart disease and cancer parallels the rise in processed food. What really happened behind the scenes was the birth of mass production of meats and other foods that revolutionized the path most foods took from planting and harvesting to the dinner table.

Low-fat diets became a part of our culture, and that belief is still well entrenched today. What is the problem with processed food? It is full of "empty" calories, which are calories with no nutritional content.

Clara Peller became famous in the 1980s in a Wendy's commercial where she emphatically asked, "Where's the beef?" Well, in this case it was "where's the nutrition?" Empty calories are saturated with enriched flour, sugar, and bad fats, and no fiber or vitamins to satisfy the body's needs. The same processed food that became commonplace in the 1950s is still prevalent today. The only exception is today's processed foods are much more concentrated with chemicals and toxins. Processed food plus chemicals is a nasty combination that quickly overloads the liver and the lymphatic system and causes overstimulation of the neurological system. Since the nervous system and the immune system function in harmony, overstimulation of these systems causes major problems for the body. Right there you have a recipe for disease. If poor dietary habits are the cause, proper dietary habits have to be part of the solution. And research supports this conclusion.[2]

The Unfolding Story That Lands at the Truth

It is only through many years of research that the association between cholesterol and heart disease has been updated and better understood. This is what the latest research is saying. Refined carbohydrates such as bread, pasta, white flour, cookies, and other sugary foods, including value meals and microwave dinners, are devoid of the vital nutrients necessary to maintain health. The body simply does not receive the proper fuel from these food sources. What happens when meal after meal is consumed that does not contain a full spectrum of vitamins and minerals? You guessed it. Nutritional deficiencies are the end result with poor health soon to follow. The belly is full, but the body is nutritionally starved. The body stores some vitamins and minerals, but most of them need to be replenished every day to maintain health.

Overconsumption of empty calories has been strongly linked with higher occurrences of cancer, thyroid problems, and diabetes, to name a few.

Here's the Bad Stuff

Excess *sugar* from processed foods is chemically converted to *cholesterol* with the help of the hormone *insulin*. From there, two things happen: cholesterol levels rise in the blood, which forces the body to store the cholesterol in the tissues as excess fat. Don't blame the body; the body is merely reacting to the conditions in which it is exposed. You may ask, isn't insulin for regulating blood sugar? Yes, that's correct. The key word here is *excess* for both insulin and cholesterol. Excess sugar in the diet causes excess insulin production. The body reacts to the excess of these guys by converting the excess sugar to cholesterol and storing it in the tissue and arteries. Notice cholesterol is produced from sugar, not fat. Dietary fat intake is important, but saturated fat does not produce cholesterol. This is only part of the story though.

Insulin is also a key player in creating *inflammation* and ultimately a host of deadly diseases. Now we're getting to the heart of the matter. Insulin, along with several other key enzymes, including Cox- two enzymes, drives the chemical conversion of sugar *and* bad fats to a nasty omega-6 fat called Arachidonic acid (AA). Remember that name because it's a big piece of the disease process. In fact, some experts now call this process "the theory of everything." Meaning, *every* chronic disease is rooted in this nasty production of inflammation. Through a long series of chemical reactions, Arachidonic acid produces an inflammatory chemical called prostaglandin E2 (PGE2). Remember this guy too. He's an even larger piece of the puzzle.

It's interesting that EPA, one the active components in fish oil, blocks this conversion of AA to PGE2 with no side effects. The benefits of fish oil will be discussed in chapter 5 and 9.

Did you catch what happened here? As if excess consumption of refined carbohydrates wasn't damaging enough, now we add damaging omega-6 fats to the list of health destroyers. Omega-6 fats are hidden in just about all of our modern foods from cooking oils to salad dressings to animal feed.

What does PGE2 do to the body?

> **PGE2** is now considered the *number one* food-induced, cancer-causing chemical on the planet.
> **PGE2** screws up the immune system and causes trauma to the brain.
> **PGE2** causes damage in the brain that is associated with bipolar disorder and depression.
> **PGE2** is strongly linked with allergies, autism, and attention deficit disorder.
> **PGE2** is strongly linked with chronic pain.

... and that is just a short list of its damaging effects.[3–4]

Even when people try to eat healthy, PGE2 rears its ugly head. "Healthy" microwave dinners seem like a better choice than a burger, fries, and a milk shake. Isn't that the common perception? These supposedly healthier choices, however, are still processed. They still contain additives, preservatives, and flavor enhancers to extend shelf life and make them taste better. But the real bad guy is the refined oils contained in these foods. Look at the long list of ingredients with words you can't pronounce. This is the first clue that chemicals have been added and good nutrition is missing.

Consuming any processed food has the potential to increase highly inflammatory PGE2. The only way around this is to eat mostly raw organic food. Instead processed food and refined carbohydrates have become and remain the staples of the American diet. Fast food is refined and highly processed, but so are 90 percent of the foods on the interior aisles of the grocery store. Processed food is full of refined sugar and bad fats that ramp up Arachidonic acid in the blood. What is happening here is simple: The more refined and processed food people eat, the more inflamed they become. The inflammation damages the lining of the arteries, causing cholesterol to collect on the damaged areas in an attempt to repair the damage. The inflammation damages the lining of the arteries long before cholesterol begins to deposit on the artery walls. Cholesterol is just an innocent bystander.

Health Tip: Processed food causes inflammation. Inflammation damages the lining of the arteries. Cholesterol sticks to the damaged arteries and forms plaque that clogs the arteries.

Commercial meat damages the arteries in a similar way. Most commercial cattle are raised on a corn and grain diet; even our restaurants advertise their meat as corn fed. Corn and grain, however, are not a natural diet for cows. They are the staple diet for commercial cattle for one reason only: it fattens the cow quickly and helps the farmer sell more cattle. The problem is that corn and grain contain the same pro-inflammatory omega-6 fat as refined carbohydrates: Arachidonic acid (AA). AA saturates the meat as it is fed to the cow, and this is the reason why red meat raises cholesterol: it is highly inflammatory. It's because of what the cows are eating. Experts call it "obese meat" for a reason.

Cows are meant to graze on grass. The meat produced by a grass-fed cow is completely different in the type of fat it contains. Grass-fed beef is rich in omega-3 fats, which are known to be anti-inflammatory. As a food source, corn and grain have a completely opposite effect on the human body and on the cow. Again the research supports this conclusion.[5,6]

There is still a disconnect between what science knows and what is communicated to the public. Even with the wealth of evidence that confirms refined carbohydrates and bad fats are causing cancer, heart disease, and many other diseases, our food guidelines still advise people to eat a low-fat diet, rich in whole grains (promoting AA and PGE2). Talk about old beliefs dying slowly. We're well into the ninetieth decade of believing this is healthy! The belief that cholesterol causes heart disease is entrenched in this theory as well. It is so evident that people are being led in the wrong direction by looking at the statistics and looking around at our citizens. My question is how much evidence do we need that we are on the wrong path when the literature clearly and repeatedly shows that grains and processed carbs are not healthy?[7]

Now that science understands the true mechanisms that cause heart disease, many prominent medical doctors are speaking out on this issue. This series of quotes, adapted from *Health and Nutrition Secrets That Can Save Your Life* by Dr. Russell Blaylock, effectively summarizes the entire situation regarding reduced-fat, high-grain diets. He says the following:

- "The average person consumes an enormous amount of cancer-stimulating fats." (AA)
- "The truly upsetting thing is that few oncologists [or doctors] tell their patients to avoid these inflammatory Omega-6 oils in their diet."
- "Trusting patients have no idea that the diet being promoted by their oncologist is actually making their cancer grow faster and metastasize."
- "AA is known to make cancer more aggressive."

Those are bold words, but there are more physicians who agree with these statements.

Dr. Dwight Lundell, a renowned cardiologist, posted this memo in an article titled *Prevent Disease* in May 2012.[8] I know this is a bit long, but I've posted key points of his commentary as a point of emphasis.

Dr. Lundell says this:

> "We physicians, with all of our training, knowledge, and authority often acquire a rather large ego that tends to make it difficult to admit we were wrong. As a heart surgeon with 25 years of experience, having performed over 5,000 open-heart surgeries, today is my day to be wrong with medical and scientific fact.
>
> I trained for many years with other prominent physicians labeled "opinion makers." Bombarded with scientific literature and continually attending continuing education seminars, we opinion makers insisted heart disease resulted from the simple fact of elevated blood cholesterol. The only accepted therapy was prescribing medications to lower cholesterol and a diet that was severely restricted in fat intake. ...Deviations from these recommendations were considered *heresy* and quite possibly could result in malpractice. These recommendations are no longer scientifically or morally defensible. Despite the fact that 25% of the population takes expensive statin medications and the fact that we have reduced fat content of our diets, more Americans will die this year of heart disease than ever before."

Here are more key points of his commentary:

- Seventy-five million Americans currently suffer from heart disease.
- Twenty million have diabetes; fifty-seven million have pre-diabetes (insulin resistance). [I believe these figures are low; other sources say it could be as high as 75 percent of the population is insulin resistant or heading in that direction.]
- These disorders are affecting younger and younger people in greater numbers. [Absolutely. This supports what I said previously.]
- Simply stated, without inflammation in the body, there is no way that cholesterol would accumulate in the wall of blood vessels. ...If we chronically expose the body to injury from toxins or foods the human body was never designed to process, a condition occurs called chronic inflammation.
- The low-fat diet recommended for years by mainstream medicine has caused injury and inflammation in our blood vessels.

Overconsumption of processed foods creates heart disease, high blood pressure, diabetes, and finally Alzheimer's disease.
- Mainstream medicine made a terrible mistake when it advised people to avoid saturated fat in favor of foods high in inflammatory omega-6 fats. We now have an epidemic of arterial inflammation leading to heart disease and other silent killers."
- He says the arteries of an inflamed person look like someone scrubbed them with sandpaper.

I respect the opinion of both Dr. Blaylock and Dr. Lundell. I could list many other quotes from cardiologists and others who are coming to the same conclusion and establishing new medical territory with their comments. When Dr. Blaylock says doctors are not talking to their patients about the dangers of inflammatory omega six oils, as a neurosurgeon with forty years of experience, I think he may have witnessed this directly when working with and referring to other specialists. Either way, taking a stand is going to step on some toes but these doctors are risking their careers to take a stand for what is right. The truth was always there, waiting to be discovered. It has just taken a long time to uncover it and acknowledge it. A change in established beliefs is happening right in front of our eyes, and we need to embrace this change with open arms. They are establishing that the world is round by essentially saying "we must acknowledge the truth." Growing pains are sometimes difficult for the ones who are establishing new territory, but truth always wins in the end.

Unhealthy Oil Number One: Trans Fats

It took forty years for science to finally prove that trans-fat is causing artery disease and another twenty years to prove that other types of fats are causing cancer. In spite of the evidence, the use of trans-fat continues in most commercial baked goods. For forty-plus years this destructive food was promoted as being healthy. I think this is one reason why so many people have a cynical attitude about changing their dietary habits. Once it becomes an accepted belief within the culture, it becomes harder to change. We were told margarine was healthier than butter and low fat was healthier than high fat. It became part of our culture. Now we are being told that was wrong after all. Changing this cultural belief is not going to be easy. The fact remains, the faster our nation abandons the low-fat, high-grain diet for the healthier alternative diet rich in anti-inflammatory omega-3 fats, the faster we will address the escalation of chronic disease. There are other factors, but this is a starting point.[9]

In case you had any doubts, here are some facts about hydrogenated oil. Most importantly, it is indigestible by the body. It has a half-life of *eight years*. In other words, it takes sixteen years for one exposure to be removed from the body.

Chemists who were manufacturing plastics discovered hydrogenated oil. They found that vegetable oil could stay solid at room temperature by injecting hydrogen ions into the oil through hydrogenation. They also learned that hydrogenation extends the shelf life of the oil almost indefinitely. Even flies won't touch it. Anything that stays in the body that long is toxic. It has to collect somewhere. That is why it collects in the arteries. Toxins are difficult for the body to break down. Thus they linger in the brain and the organs, causing damage and disease. Most of the damage comes from inflammatory reactions in the organs and the arteries.

Unhealthy Oils, Two and Three: Vegetable Oils and Seed Oils

Regarding other types of non-hydrogenated vegetable oils and seed oils, the literature is full of medical references indicating that these oils produce Arachidonic acid (AA) in the body with the help of our old buddies, insulin and cox 2 enzymes. AA in turn produces the nasty chemical PGE2, which is a major cause of cancer. You've heard of them: canola oil, safflower oil, peanut oil, cottonseed oil, and palm oil—they all contain a high amount of inflammatory omega-6 fat. Cottonseed oil alone has a 234:1 ratio of bad omega-6 oil to good omega-3 oil. In the petroleum world that's called "high octane." In this case high octane is throwing fuel on an inflammation process that turns deadly. One would think this would have resulted in restriction of their use, but that is not the case at all. Non-hydrogenated vegetable oil is still widely used as a replacement for hydrogenated oil in many foods. These "heart-healthy" oils are loaded with inflammation-producing omega-6 oils that drive AA to produce PGE2. This is a significant portion of the explosion in chronic disease. Add in the explosion of toxins in foods and the environment, and we truly have the equivalent of gasoline on a fire.

This is even more evidence of the disconnect between science and public perception. Now we see evidence of the disconnect coming from the authority figures in medicine - the opinion makers that drive policy and research. Why are we not hearing more about this? I'm convinced this is purely a result of the depth of the fat-restriction movement and the fast pace of our society that caters toward convenience foods. And the stubborn refusal of the opinion makers to change the guidelines that perpetuate this misguided movement.

On one hand, the public cannot be faulted for lacking awareness of the dangers of fat-restricted diets. On the other hand, science cannot be completely at fault for people's dietary choices. Someone must bridge the gap so science and the public are on the same page. The only way that will happen is for more and more authority figures who know the truth to talk about it, write about it, and educate the masses. By the way, this is the one-hundredth monkey syndrome that starts with one, then another, and then another. By the time the one-hundredth monkey develops the habit, it spreads to every monkey. No, we're not monkeys, but the concept applies to humans.

Health Tip: For healthier cooking, use olive oil or coconut oil. Always cook using the lowest heat setting possible and increase cooking times if necessary.

The simple truth is we still have some work to do on this topic to get where we need to be. The food industry still believes that omega-6 oils are heart healthy. The food companies still advertise their oils as heart healthy, and they are routinely used in prepared foods in grocery stores and restaurants.

You Have the Power

The food guidelines have changed very little over the past thirty to forty years. I think the engine that drives change in this case is going to be *you*, the consumer. As more people become educated on the damaging effects of these oils, you will see the food makers follow suit and remove them from their products.

The same thing is happening with high-fructose corn syrup (HFCS). Some breads, pastries, and condiments are labeled "contains no high-fructose corn syrup." There seems to be an underground movement that is influencing food makers to remove HFCS from their products, even though it is not a banned substance. This could be another instance of consumer demand influencing product manufacturing.

In the meantime, I have come to the conclusion after reviewing enough data that people are still dying of malnutrition, even in this modern age. And there are people dying from advanced heart disease who are seemingly doing the right thing by exercising regularly and trying to eat right based on what they know. They are eating but still starving their cells by consuming too many foods with empty calories.

The hidden danger of junk foods that are so prevalent today is they are empty calories with no nutritional value. A belly full of pizza will give you a good dose of fat and protein, and a bunch of synthetic chemicals, with little else. The belly is full and we feel satisfied, but we still don't have a good balance of vitamins, antioxidants, and good omega-3 fats to satisfy the body's needs. Fast food is a common staple of our culture. A quick run through the drive-through is a mainstay for many busy families. Instead of subsidizing the disease-care industry, we would be well served to subsidize health-enhancing habits, such as balanced meals that contain ample quantities of vegetables, quality protein, and good fats.

As we will see in the next chapter, consuming trans- fat is one portion of the mystery connecting fat intake to vascular disease and stroke. It points to inflammation as the primary cause of chronic illness and chronic pain.

The Natural Course of History

We are making progress, but there is a long way to go. Change is difficult when the long-held belief is grounded in things that are not true. I look at the situation with a lighter perspective. If we can change people's long-held beliefs about diet, we have 50 percent of the battle won. We can also look at progress from a historical perspective. The belief that the world was flat prevailed for centuries before the philosopher Pythagoras proposed a bold new theory in sixth century BC: he said the earth was not flat, it's round. It took another 150 years of rejection, debate, and criticism before the theory became common knowledge. When I look at it from this perspective, we must be right on schedule.

CHAPTER 4

Understanding Cause and Effect

> What makes toxins "toxic" is the fact that they rev up free radical production and promote inflammation.
>
> —David Perlmutter, MD

As the quote above suggests, we know toxic chemicals cause inflammation in the tissues, organs, and joints of the body. From here it gets more complicated. Inflammation produces free radicals. Free radicals produce more inflammation. It becomes a vicious cycle. Inflammation, in turn, causes chronic pain syndromes and many of the chronic diseases that are running rampant through our society. Remember those statistics from chapter 2 regarding chronic pain? OTC pain medications are called NSAIDs, which stands for non-steroidal anti-inflammatory drugs. These medications are used to address inflammation, but are they really addressing the root cause of the inflammation? And are there safer ways to address inflammation than through the use of NSAIDs? As we have seen, short-term pain relief often comes at the expense of destroying your liver and kidneys.

In my quest to find answers, I reviewed volumes of research. I wanted to find out what the current research says about inflammation. As I did, I had to ask myself some challenging questions. If the root cause of pain is inflammation, is it possible to go right to the source of the inflammation and stop it before it causes damage, but do so without damaging side effects? Is it possible that other classes of drugs are in some way addressing the same damaging effects of inflammation that cause the body to break down, but not addressing the root cause? As I studied the sources of inflammation, I became more and more convinced that the current research is on the right track. I learned that inflammation must be an important topic because the PubMed database is full of references relating to this subject.

> **Side note:** PubMed, also called the National Center for Biotechnology Information, is a free online search engine that posts medical research articles. It contains over twenty-six million references related to any medical or health topic. In the course of writing this book, I wanted to see how many references would come up if I did a simple but nonspecific search using the word *inflammation.* A generic search for "inflammation" brought up 538,355 research articles. I thought, "Whoa, that's pretty impressive." So I refined my search to "inflammation and cancer," which brought up 61,568 articles. Hmm, that's even more interesting: over sixty-one thousand references linking inflammation to cancer. I refined the search again, this time to "inflammation and oxidative stress." This search brought up 22,672 articles. I knew I was on the right track. This volume of data would not exist without purpose. What is even more impressive is how fast these numbers are growing. At one point, when I repeated the search for inflammation, the number of published articles had grown by over three thousand articles ... in only two months. The numbers for every search had grown significantly though. I had to go back and update my numbers multiple times.

These searches prove inflammation is not just a new kid on the block that was recently discovered. Quite the contrary, inflammation is a topic that has been and continues to be well researched.

If this information is so important, why don't we hear more about this invisible, silent killer? Wouldn't you want to know if there was a killer on the loose that could harm you or your family? I would. As I reflect on possible answers to that question, I am considering many possibilities. Unless you're a medical professional, you would have no reason to scour the PubMed database in search of these articles. We still rely heavily on medical professionals to provide the information we need to know. They serve as the messengers. Other than the occasional article that hits newsstands or a five-minute segment on the local TV news, scientific information like this is not newsworthy.

Chronic Inflammation: What Is It and Where Does It Come From?

The role of the immune system is not strictly to fight infection. It also initiates the repair of aged or damaged tissue. This is a key point to understand in acute versus chronic inflammation. Acute inflammation is a natural part of the healing process that follows tissue injury, in which the immune system regulates tissue repair; for example, following the sprain of a twisted ankle. Its progression would look something like this:

Figure 2.

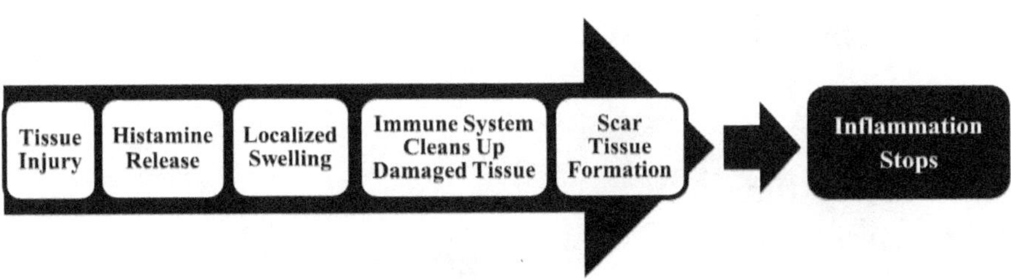

Chronic inflammation is more complex than just acute swelling. Chronic inflammation becomes systemic—it travels throughout the body. It is a silent, destructive process that suppresses the immune response that cleans up the original injury, effectively prolonging the resolution of the original source of the injury or infection (the end point). This allows the immune system to target healthy tissue, causing tissue damage and disease. In other words, chronic inflammation hinders the body's ability to repair and heal properly because it has no end point.

Figure 3 below visualizes the difference between acute and chronic inflammation.

Figure 3.

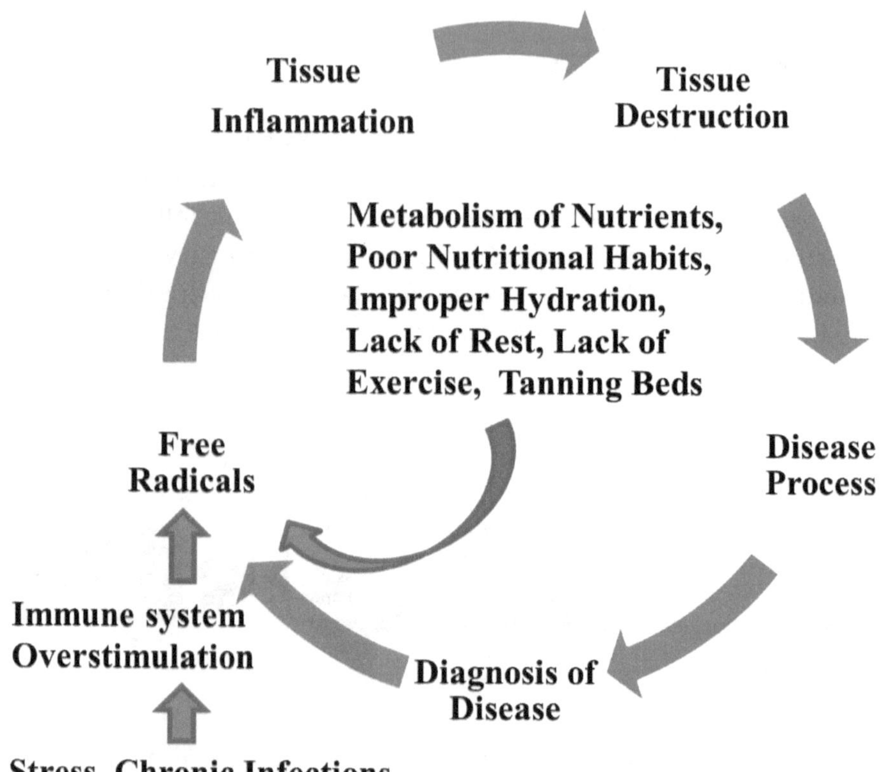

The data suggests that hormones produced during stress combined with inflammation from the diet causes the progression to chronic inflammation.[1] Stress hormones hinder the ability of the immune response to fight infection and repair injury. Please understand the importance of this scientific discovery. This is a key piece of information that points us to the root cause of chronic disease.

A perpetually stimulated immune system causes degenerative disease and cancer. Let me repeat that: a perpetually stimulated immune system causes degenerative disease and cancer. We know this beyond any shadow of a doubt. The importance of this message is beyond critical. With understanding comes wisdom.

Illnesses such as heart disease and cancer are a result of this vicious cycle. For those with a clinical background, the literature says that pro-inflammatory cytokines are one class of immune cells that become overactive and trigger the disease process. The grand design of the body just responds to the conditions to which it's exposed. If you don't like the response, change the input. If stress and diet initiate chronic inflammation, the first thing that changes the input to the immune system is to lower your stress and improve your diet.

Without an "end point," chronic inflammation can spread quickly through the body causing serious damage. Scientists have known for many years that stress plays a key role in the disease process, but they didn't understand the mechanism behind it. Now they know beyond any doubt that this is a primary factor that drives the disease process. Pair prolonged periods of poor dietary habits with prolonged periods of stress and you have a recipe for disaster.

Chronic Infections

Chronic infections such as Lyme disease act in a similar fashion as traumatic injury. Initially, the immune system releases a massive assault against the infection. Under normal circumstances the immune system cleans up the bacteria and then the immune cells dissipate. However, the bacteria that causes Lyme disease is so potent that the immune system often has a very difficult time fighting off the infection. This allows the invasion to progress deeper into the body, but the progression is magnified if the person is under emotional stress and is already inflamed.[2] As the infection becomes chronic the body continues to release immune cells, but over time the infection overwhelms the immune system, causing the immune response to attack its own tissue. Early detection is the key to overcoming this type of chronic infection. This is a case where antibiotics may be necessary to help the body overcome the infection and prevent it from becoming chronic. However, decreasing stress and improving the diet are also very important in sustaining a healthy body.

Free Radicals: The Basics

> When an electron vibrates, the whole earth shakes.
>
> —Deepak Chopra

Free radicals play a key role in chronic inflammation. Before I get to that, here are some key points about free radicals:

The atom is the basic building block for everything in the universe, including the human body. Atoms are composed of an inner nucleus of protons and neutrons, with electrons suspended in orbit around the nucleus. A free radical is an unpaired electron that is displaced from the atom and circulates within the body. (See figure 4 below).

Figure 4.

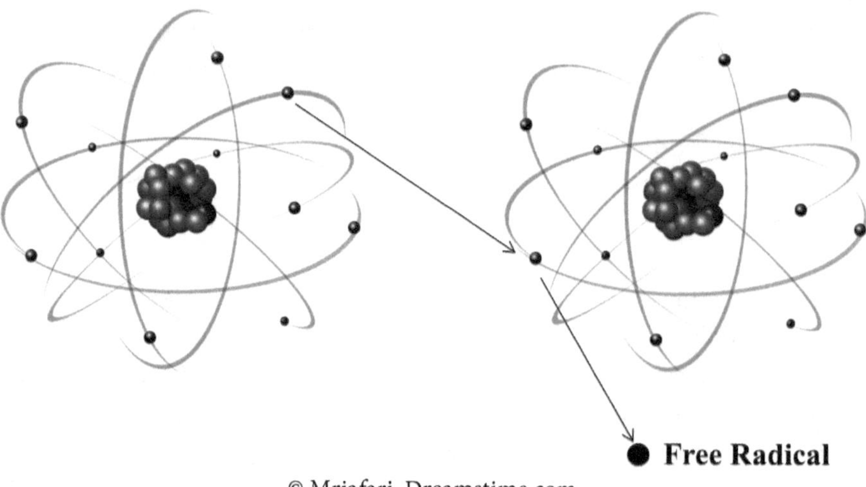

Much like water eroding rock, free radicals cause damage to surrounding cells and tissues. Free radicals are especially damaging to the inner lining of the arteries and organs. Think about Jim Fixx when you read that sentence.

My PubMed searches indicate that free radicals and inflammation are a central theme of the research data on the cause of chronic disease—the same conclusions appear over and over, in study after study. The research is clear about their destructive power. The body is under a continuous assault from these little particles with the power of a nuclear bomb. They are constantly being produced so the body is under a constant threat. We now know there are many factors that cause free radicals to be produced. The most common sources of free radicals are poor diet, stress, environmental toxins, ultraviolet radiation (tanning beds), X-rays, low magnesium intake (vitamin and mineral deficiencies), and immune system reactions. Even vigorous exercise generates large amounts of free radicals. Some of these factors will be discussed later, but we don't have to talk about all of them to get the big picture. Free-radical damage can be prevented before it reaches full-blown disease through lifestyle changes.

It's amazing that something so small can be so destructive. The damage to the tissues is a silent process that can take months or even years to appear. By the time you feel the effects, critical damage has already begun.

In summary:

The fundamental, underlying theme in nearly all disease is inflammation (there's your common denominator for all diseases, the theory of everything). Where does it come from? By far the most abundant source of inflammation is from free radicals. Toxins produce them, the body produces them. We can't escape them but we can manage them to minimize the damage.

As I describe this process, can you visualize free radical production in your mind? A free radical doesn't wander aimlessly. It has a mission: it constantly looks for a mate. Since the free radical has a negative charge, it is always in competition with other electrons. As electrons migrate through the body, they bump into other cells, knocking other electrons into free circulation much like a bowling ball hitting bowling pins. Science has called this process "oxidative stress." Each time the electron bumps into healthy tissue, the tissue becomes damaged, much like a bullet hitting a target. It doesn't take a rocket scientist to figure out that something serious is going to happen if the process continues to fire, just like an automatic rifle.

Once free radicals are produced, they continue to damage tissue throughout the body until something absorbs the electrons and repairs the damage that was created in their wake. That "something" is called an antioxidant. The job of an antioxidant is to protect the body from free-radical damage by absorbing them from circulation. The most common antioxidants are vitamin A, vitamin C, vitamin E, selenium, and the most powerful of all antioxidants, glutathione. (Vitamins and supplements will be covered in more detail in chapter 9.)

Even though there are many sources of free radicals, the most abundant source comes from within the cells of your body through the metabolism of nutrients. *As your metabolism increases, so does the production of free radicals.* How do you protect yourself from them? Your defense against free radicals is threefold:

1. Limit their production.
2. Neutralize them when they are produced.
3. Repair the damage to the cells and tissue.

I'll cover these later in greater detail. For now just know that these three things are accomplished by proper lifestyle habits, especially by maintaining a proper diet and through nutritional supplementation.

Dr. Blaylock gives an excellent summary of free radicals in *Health and Nutrition Secrets*:[3] (emphasis added).

> We now know that aging, as well as degenerative diseases [seven of the top ten causes of death listed in chapter two] are the result of a lifetime of assaults on our cells. Medical science has realized that *all* diseases occur on a cellular and even a molecular level. The process that results in what we call "aging" is slowly being understood. For example, we now know that from the time we are first formed in our mother's womb, our cells are producing destructive particles called free radicals, and over a lifetime these free radicals chip away at our cells, like water wearing away a stone, until the cells are so weakened they begin to malfunction. We call this process aging, and in extreme cases *degenerative disease.*

Even though the research on free radicals is very detailed I have tried to simplify things to make it more understandable. From my perspective, we are in the midst of an epidemic, but this time it's not about the spread of infection. It's inflammation.

In case you are questioning whether or not this is another half-truth like the fabled health benefits of margarine, the researchers have it right as to the *cause* of these chronic diseases. The fact that one source can cause so many problems tells me this is an epidemic unlike anything we have seen before. If we know inflammation is the root cause of chronic disease, what can be done to address this epidemic?

For example; can we prevent free-radical damage using only drugs and surgery (the technology model)? To my knowledge there are no drugs that accomplish this goal right now. Oh, there are prescription drugs that address inflammation. Cox 2 inhibitor drugs were released to the market many years ago for this purpose. The problem was the side effects. Cox 2 inhibitors can cause severe and sometimes fatal intestinal bleeding. In fact the problem was so severe that one of the drugs was pulled from the market. Cox 2 inhibitors still don't address the free radicals though. They are addressing the downstream effects of inflammation just like the OTC NSAIDS mentioned earlier.

In the future there may be new classes of drugs that address free radicals without side effects. My fear would be that the side effects from these drugs might be more destructive than the free radicals themselves, just as we have experienced with Cox 2 inhibitors. Why wait for that unknown day in the future when we know *now* how to address free radicals through diet and supplementation? We know how to accomplish this; it just takes education and lifestyle changes to do it.

In summary: we limit production of free radicals by keeping a healthy environment inside the cells. Stress, poor diet, and extreme physical activity are by far the biggest generators of free radicals, so this is the foundation from which to begin. Let's cover each of these in more detail.

Free Radicals From Exercise

You mean to tell me that exercise produces destructive free radicals? The answer is yes. As your body produces energy inside the cells from the digestion of nutrients, free radicals are released into the system. This also means that exercise, or any activity that causes you to breathe harder or sweat, increases free-radical production. It was once thought that cardiovascular exercise was most beneficial for fat burning once you went beyond the first thirty minutes. The theory was the body transitioned from burning glucose to fat to produce energy after about thirty minutes. This was supposed to equate to better weight loss and a better workout. While this is true from a purely physiological perspective, the free radicals that are generated in long-duration exercise can have a detrimental effect on a person's health.

It is now becoming widely accepted that short-term, high-intensity training (also called interval training) is more beneficial for the body because it minimizes free-radical production and stimulates sustained growth-hormone release from the pituitary gland. Exercising is extremely beneficial in moderation, especially when coupled with an anti-inflammatory diet rich in omega-3 fatty acids and high antioxidant intake.

Limiting free-radical production involves "healthy" exercise.[4] Notice, this does not say that exercise is bad. It says there is a healthy way to exercise that maximizes the benefit and limits the risk. One of the world's leading authorities on the benefits of exercise is Dr. Ken Cooper. Dr. Cooper founded aerobics as a form of exercise in the early 1970s. He states that the main goal of exercise is to strengthen the body and ultimately make a person healthier. Yet Dr. Cooper has clearly identified intense, prolonged exercise as a risk factor for producing large amounts of free radicals, which are associated with increased risk of degenerative disease and shortened life span. He discovered over time that his most dedicated patients (to aerobics) were the ones who were dying of advanced heart disease. Aerobics is supposed to make you healthier, not make you die prematurely. That's not the way it's supposed to work.

The risk of damaging the body through exercise should be taken seriously by everyone from trained athletes to casual participants. Can you imagine the number of free radicals that are produced by professional athletes during a football or basketball game? Or from a farmer working in the fields? We are all subject to the effects of free radicals.

Dr. Cooper says the only way to counter the effects of free radicals is by supplementing with antioxidants on a daily basis—especially *before* exercise. (See chapter nine for a more detailed list of antioxidants). This is the only way to get the full benefit of exercise and minimize the potential damage that can occur if precautions are not taken seriously. This updates the previous belief that no food should be consumed within two hours of exercise; otherwise, the food may not digest properly. It just needs to be the right type of nutrients.

In summary, experts now suggest that we should never exercise without consuming antioxidants beforehand and never exercise on a completely empty stomach. Drinking a protein smoothie, containing vitamins and antioxidants, thirty to forty-five minutes before exercise is the best way to limit free-radical damage. This will provide adequate fuel for the cells and antioxidants to absorb free radicals produced by the exercise. Experts also recommend short-term, high-intensity exercise, such as interval training for aerobic benefit. Obviously this will depend on your fitness level, but fifteen to twenty minutes of high-intensity exercise is better for the body than sixty minutes of prolonged, medium-intensity exercise. This will maximize the aerobic benefit while minimizing the damage from free-radical production during the exercise. Short-term, high-intensity exercise has been shown to produce higher sustained levels of human growth hormone (HGH) after exercise. HGH is associated with healthy cell reproduction and decreases the effects of aging.

Stress and Free Radicals

No discussion of free-radical damage would be complete without addressing the effects of stress on the body. In this case, I am talking specifically about emotional stress. Neuroscientists have proven that emotions have specific stimulatory effects on the body. We know through these studies that the autonomic nervous system, which controls all of the subconscious actions of the body—including heartbeat, digestion, detoxification, immune system reactions, brain chemistry, etc.—is strongly stimulated by emotional stress. Stress produces large amounts of chemicals and hormones that are dumped into the bloodstream (cortisol, epinephrine, and norepinephrine). Prolonged overproduction of these hormones has a very damaging effect on the body, especially the immune system. These are the stress hormones that overstimulate the immune system with no end point. Remember what stimulation of metabolism does to free-radical production? Yes, it increases it.

The following list contains some of the documented effects of prolonged stress:

1. Stress suppresses the immune system.
2. Stress reduces blood flow and oxygen supply to the organs and tissues, including the brain.
3. Stress impairs gene expression and healing.
4. Stress increases inflammation (PGE2).
5. Stress increases free radicals.

Stress is generated in the brain but ripples throughout the entire body through chemical production. The chart below gives a partial list of chemicals produced by specific emotions and the effects of those chemicals on the body:

Figure 5.Stress-induced chemical production

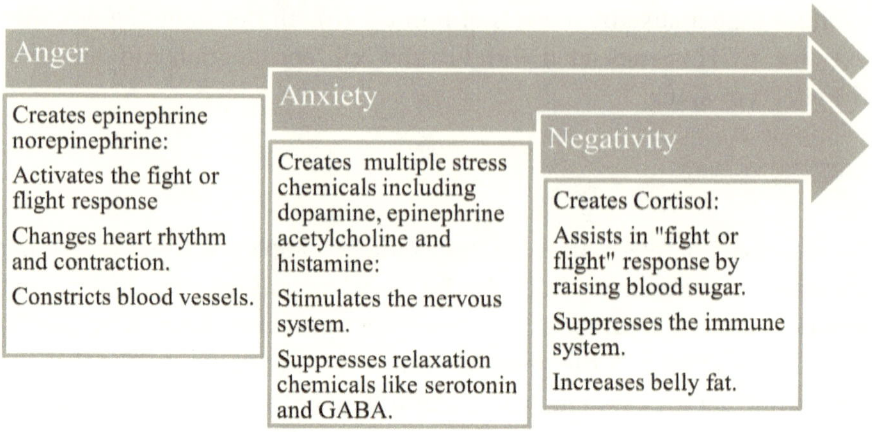

Anger

Creates epinephrine norepinephrine:

Activates the fight or flight response

Changes heart rhythm and contraction.

Constricts blood vessels.

Anxiety

Creates multiple stress chemicals including dopamine, epinephrine acetylcholine and histamine:

Stimulates the nervous system.

Suppresses relaxation chemicals like serotonin and GABA.

Negativity

Creates Cortisol:

Assists in "fight or flight" response by raising blood sugar.

Suppresses the immune system.

Increases belly fat.

The key to understand here is that emotions stimulate chemical production in the body. Worry and anxiety stimulate digestion even if there is no food in the gut to be digested. Anger increases heart rate and blood pressure even if the person is sitting on the couch watching TV. Hostility produces multiple chemicals that can alter immune system function, raise blood pressure, and stimulate digestion all at the same time.

Many times, when an individual is going through a stressful situation, it is not just a one-time thing. In fact, most stressful situations are ongoing. What we think about today we are likely to think about tomorrow and the next day and the next day, and so on.

We think with feeling. This is what gives situations their meaning. We feel angry, we feel panic, we feel hostility, we feel joy, and we feel gratitude. We feel emotions in the mind *and* the body. Emotions give meaning to the circumstances of life. Emotions help the body adapt itself for survival at that very moment. It does not matter if the emotions are coming from the memory of a past event or from a present experience. The fear and adrenaline rush from being chased by a bear is exactly the same as the memory of being chased by the bear. The physiology is exactly the same. Psychologists refer to this as the "fight or flight" response. The memory of an event has the potential to have a greater impact on the body because the memory becomes recorded in the subconscious mind. The memory is there in the subconscious part of the brain. It activates the survival response even when the person is not actively thinking about the event that caused it.

Health Tip: Emotions have a powerful input to the body. Past emotions can override the normal function of your body in the present, which hinders the healing of the body.

There is actually a scientific term for this phenomenon. The term, originally proposed by M. T. Morter Jr., DC, is called SEMO, the abbreviation for subconscious emotional memory override.[5] Everyone has experienced SEMO at different times in their lives, especially after stressful events. SEMO has a powerful effect on the body's ability to heal and self-regulate by exciting the nervous system long after the original event occurred.

When metabolism becomes stimulated, either through dietary toxins or by emotions, the body produces free radicals in response to that increased metabolism. We must keep in mind that God has hardwired the body to function this way. If we are being threatened, it doesn't matter if a person is running from a bear or coping with an abusive relationship. The survival response and its corresponding chemical production are still hardwired into the body. The emotions are connecting with the physical body for the purpose of survival.

The last thing we need if we're running from a bear is for our heart rate to decrease. The muscles in our arms and legs need that raised heart rate to deliver blood, oxygen, and nutrients. In this instance, we *want* to have a higher blood pressure and a high pulse rate to pump blood into our muscles. Escaping the bear is the high priority at that moment, not digesting food or fighting infection. The entire body is redirected to survive the crisis. Few people, however, are truly running from a bear. They are adapting their bodies for survival in everyday life. And this adaptation is what causes problems.

One Duke University study is a classic example of SEMO. In the study, researchers found that a large percentage of participants had heart disease without the traditional risk factors: obesity, smoking, diabetes, hypertension, high cholesterol, sedentary lifestyles, etc. There had to be a cause even in the absence of the traditional risk factors. So researchers dug deeper. The only common ground among the participants was that they all shared significant hurtful events from the past in which they had not expressed forgiveness.

The researchers concluded that suppressed anger, hostility, and depression were the key predictors for heart disease in these individuals. Participants who identified chronic anger and hostility with past events had significantly higher blood levels of a chemical called C-reactive protein; C-reactive protein is a strong producer of inflammation.

Anger → C-reactive protein → inflammation → damaged artery lining → heart disease

This study clearly challenges the traditional notion of cholesterol as the cause of heart disease. If you remember, heart disease is now the number one cause of mortality in the United States and a rising cause of death in many other industrialized nations. This study would suggest that there are a lot of people who are suppressing hostility. It also supports other studies that show stress as a producer of inflammation.[6]

Other studies have shown that expectant moms with high levels of the stress hormone cortisol (produced when the mom is stressed) give birth to babies who have high cortisol levels. Cortisol adapts the body for stress by raising blood sugar, but it also lowers resistance to infection and causes increased belly fat. The key point to understand here is the mother's stress is programing the unborn child for blood sugar issues (diabetes) before they are born. The diabetic condition may show up later in life but the precipitating factors were initiated in utero. Even cells of an unborn baby can have SEMO memory patterns. Dr. Bruce Lipton, who I mentioned in chapter one, has some fascinating research on this subject - research that has extreme implications on when the origin of disease actually occurs.

The mind-body connection is powerful. I could write an entire book on that subject alone. Even the Bible admonishes us to guard our heart and guard our thoughts (which lead to our emotional state).

> Above everything else, guard your heart because from it flows the springs of life.
>
> —Proverbs 4:23 NIV

CHAPTER 5

Inflammation and Its Impact on the Cells

A deeper understanding of inflammation's destructive effect on the cells is vital to understanding the cause of chronic disease. The concepts explained in this chapter will be used throughout the remainder of this book.

Cells: Building Blocks of Life

To fully understand the effect of inflammation on the body, we must first understand the basics about the cell and its surrounding environment. The building blocks that collectively form the unique and wonderful person you are essentially equal a massive collection of cells glued together by a substance called the extra-cellular matrix. Collectively, as we look at how the cells cluster together and count them one by one, we would see that your body contains over seventy trillion cells.

Looking deep inside the cell reveals an even larger cluster of atoms that are formed together in a cohesive unit, held together by forces similar to that of a magnet. The forces are invisible, but we know they exist through the laws of quantum physics.

Considering the fact that all cells are made of clusters of atoms, here are some intriguing questions to ponder: How does a cell know what to do in the body if they are merely clusters of atoms? How does a muscle cell know that it is indeed a muscle cell and not a cell of a gland or an organ? Is it programming from DNA or something deeper? What is the difference between a healthy cell and a diseased cell? Yes, we know that cells have different tissue types, but what is it that makes them different when they have the same atoms that serve as building blocks to form the cell? The atoms are exactly the same in a healthy cell as they are in a diseased cell. For now I'll call it grand design. I'll let you think about these questions as you read through the remainder of this chapter.

Different cells carry out different actions depending on where the cell is located. Cells of a gland produce hormones. Cells of a muscle produce movement, etc. It can be said that healthy cells produce a healthy body. We live and die by the proper function of the cells.

Every structure in the body is built by grand design that serves a purpose. Nothing is left to chance in the body. There is no greater evidence of that grand design than in the structure of the cells. The illustration in figure 6 is an enlarged picture of the outer portion of the cell, the cell membrane, and the inside of a cell.

Figure 6. The cell membrane and the inside of a cell

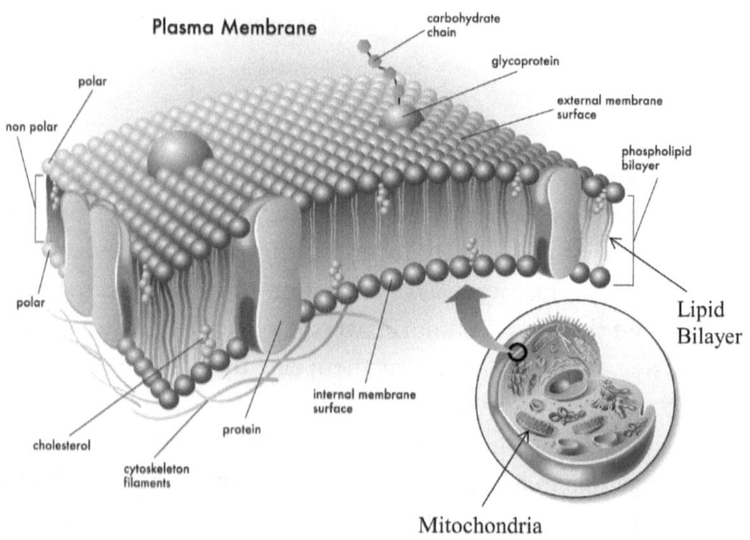

© Rob3000 | Dreamstime.com

By far, the two most important components of your cells are the outer cell membrane (magnified) and the mitochondria inside the cell (arrow on the bottom). Both serve a vital role in keeping you healthy. Why? These are the first cell components that are damaged by inflammation and free radicals. This is a key point in understanding the importance of quality fat intake in the diet, which will be discussed later in this chapter. These factors all tie together and dictate whether your cells are healthy or unhealthy.

The Cell Membrane: Good Fats Form Healthy Cells

The cell membrane is the outer portion that surrounds the cell. That means there are seventy trillion cell membranes clustered together to form your body. This outer membrane is made of small beads of fat (lipids) that are connected in a chain as illustrated in figure 6. The cell membrane is also called the *lipid bilayer* because the beads are stacked together to form two rows. Don't be confused about the lipid bilayer and the cell membrane. They mean the same thing.

What may seem like an insignificant part of the cell actually has an abundance of activity that is vital to the body. The membrane allows nutrients to pass through to the inside of the cell and serve as a source of fuel. Just as the engine in your car produces exhaust, waste products are generated inside the cell and must be expelled. The cell membrane must be fluid (flexible) enough to allow the exchange of nutrients and waste products. Any damage to the cell membrane from poor diet or inflammation will disrupt this exchange and place additional stress on the cells. Free radicals are produced if this exchange is not executed properly, which can cause damage to every functional part of the body. (This is much like the engine in your car misfiring if the fuel is not burned efficiently.) The more fluid the cell membrane, the better the cells respond to the hormones and the better the cell functions overall. Table three is an illustration of the most common sources of dietary fat that make up the cell membrane.

Table 3.

Table A.

Fat	Fluidity
Trans Fats (Hydrogenated oils)	Least Fluid
Saturated Fats (Animal Fats)	↓
Monounsaturated Fats (Olive Oil)	↓
Polyunsaturated Fats (Black Current, Flax, Walnut, Evening Primrose)	↓
EPA (from fish oil)	↓
DHA (from fish oil)	Most Fluid

The cell membrane is primarily made of lipids. Some of the lipids come from cholesterol produced in the liver. Most of the lipids come from fats in the diet. The quality of fats in the diet determines the quality of the cell membranes throughout the body. The goal in balancing dietary fat intake is to get the predominance of your fat from the sources listed inside the bracket in table three.

While a variety of fat sources is beneficial, fish oil is the best source of omega-3 fats EPA and DHA. These are the active components of fish oil. EPA is the *anti-inflammatory* component of fish oil; DHA is the *brain-building* component of fish oil that also makes up the majority of the cell membrane. The body does not manufacture these guys so they must be obtained in the diet. The best dietary sources of EPA and DHA are derived through fresh, cold-water fish, especially salmon, tuna, mackerel, and sardines.

(*Please take special note of the discussion in chapter eight on precautions related to fish consumption.)

Flax seed and flax oil also supply omega 3's but not in the form of EPA and DHA.

It is a sad reality that some sources of fish are now considered unsafe for human consumption. In the absence of pure sources of fish, the only safe alternative is to take purified fish oil in supplement form.

Over my years in clinical practice, I have often encountered questions from patients regarding omega-3 oils. Here is a summary of those questions:

1. **Can I take flax seed oil as a replacement for fish oil since I am a vegetarian?**

   No. Flax seed oil does not contain EPA and DHA. It contains an 18-carbon fat called ALA. To get the benefit of EPA and DHA, the body must convert ALA to EPA and DHA in the liver. Unfortunately, for most people the conversion of ALA to EPA is only about 20 percent efficient; the conversion of ALA to DHA is only about 3 percent efficient. *This means it's nearly impossible to get enough ALA to provide a therapeutic dose of EPA and DHA. For vegetarians the amount of flax oil required to obtain a therapeutic dose would be quite large and possibly unhealthy. Some studies have linked high doses of ALA to a higher incidence of prostate cancer as well as interrupting the fat content of the brain in depression related illness.[1] Lower doses of ALA (100-300mg) have been shown to have a protective effect against cancer. For now, it is safe to assume ALA in moderation does provide significant health benefits, especially the lignans from ground flax seed. Lignans are similar to the fiber in other vegetables that acts as an antioxidant.

2. **I can't take fish oil. When I take it, I seem to burp it up for hours.**
   In my experience, burping fish oil happens because (a) the fish oil you are taking has some contaminants in it, or (b) your body is oxidizing the fish oil after you take it.
   Make sure the oil you are using is purified to remove harmful contaminants (or at least tested for impurities). Unfortunately, many of the oceans where fish are harvested can be contaminated with PCBs (polychlorinated biphenyls) and heavy metals, such as lead and mercury. This issue resulted in a recent lawsuit filed against ten supplement companies that produce fish oil, alleging that their oils were contaminated with PCBs. Distillation can remove these contaminants but at a high cost. I believe this is the reason many companies do not distill their oil before selling it.
   Also, fish oil is inherently unstable, meaning it can oxidize very easily, even in the presence of light shining through the bottle. Look for a product that has at least ten IUs of vitamin E per gram of oil. The vitamin E is there to stabilize the oil and not necessarily for your daily nutritional intake. You can add extra vitamin E as you take the oil, but this still does not assure the oil has not oxidized.

3. **How much fish oil should I take?**
   Dosage recommendations in the literature are pretty inconsistent. I like the recommendations from Barry Sears, PhD, in his book *Toxic Fat: When Good Fat Turns Bad:*

Condition	Amount of fish oil needed
No chronic disease/pain	2.5 grams/day
Overweight, type 2 diabetes, heart disease, or before starting a weight loss program	5 grams/day
Chronic joint pain	7.5 grams /day
Neurological disease	10 grams/day

- Please note: **Do not take this much fish oil without an ample supply of antioxidants and making sure the oil is purified to remove contaminants.** Fish oil will oxidize when exposed to free radicals inside the body. The damage that can result from not following this recommendation can be severe. Everyone has at least some free radical activity, which can readily oxidize the oil as it is digested. What was once of great benefit now becomes a potential source of cancer.

To this point, antioxidants prevent oxidation (damage) to the oil and, therefore, maximize the benefit of taking it. The easy way to remember the vitamins that fall in the antioxidant category, think of the acronym "ACES:"

- A = vitamin A (minimum 3000 IU)
- C = vitamin C (minimum 150 mg)
- E = vitamin E (minimum 400 IU)
- S = selenium (minimum 50 μg)

Other helpful antioxidants include:

- CoQ10 (minimum 100 mg)
- Alpha lipoic acid (minimum 50 mg)
- Acetyl-L-carnitine (minimum 50 mg)

These nutrients are potent antioxidants that protect the cells from free radicals and assist the cells in absorbing and utilizing nutrients. This protects the mitochondria from damage.

The message to take home is this: we must consume fats, but as consumers we must distinguish between good fats and bad fats when making choices. The type of fat one consumes is equally as important as the amount of fat. Again, processed food contains mostly harmful omega 6 fats that produce Arachidonic acid. Hopefully after reading this far you know that health can't be sustained while eating a diet of burgers, doughnuts, and pizza; common food in today's society.

Some Omega-6 Oils Are Good

It should be noted that some omega 6 oils are actually healthy. Everyone should consume a minimum of 100 mg of the healthy omega-6 fat GLA. Common sources are black current seed oil, borage oil, and evening primrose oil. GLA from evening primrose oil is especially beneficial to women who experience cramping and bloating during their monthly cycles because of its anti-inflammatory and hormone-balancing effects. To be clear, GLA is not the same as the bad omega-6 fat I discussed before called Arachidonic acid. AA causes inflammation that leads to cancer. GLA aids in decreasing inflammation and enhancing cell function.

Cell-to-Cell Communication

One more thing about the lipid bilayer: it is also a very good conductor of electrical signals passing between the cells. This means the cells literally talk to each other, another example of grand design. Cell membranes built with bad fats cannot talk to each other efficiently. Communication between body parts is yet another vital factor that keeps you healthy. If an organ cannot communicate with the brain or the brain cannot communicate with an organ, it causes serious disruption in the body.

Health Tip: Saturated fats from animal sources and hydrogenated oils clog up cell membranes making them rigid and inefficient at conducting information.

The human brain is composed of nearly 70 percent fat, and the body's nerves have a coating around them called myelin that is made of mostly fat. This fat in our brain cells, nerves, and other cells conducts electrical and chemical information throughout the body. Organs and tissues literally talk to each other by sending electrical signals from one cell to the next. The danger of fat restriction or diets with the wrong type of fat is significant. Saturated fat from a diet of junk food causes the cell membranes to clog up, which restricts passage of nutrients into the cells, restricts passage of waste products from within the cells, and blocks proper cell communication. That is why it's called membrane fluidity because the membrane must be fluid enough to allow for exchange of nutrients and waste products, as well as enable the electrical signals for cell communication. Without the electrical transmission of cell communication and rapid exchange of nutrients, proper cell activity is disrupted, resulting in production of free radicals and cell death.

Receptors: The Key to Unlocking the Cells

Hormones and neurotransmitters are chemical messengers. Examples of hormones are thyroid hormones, hormones from the pancreas like insulin, and sex hormones, such as estrogen or testosterone. Examples of neurotransmitters are serotonin and epinephrine. Chemical messengers send signals to the cells to carry out specific actions, such as regulating blood sugar and blood pressure. The hormones and neurotransmitters have specific locations on the cell membrane where they receive the signal unique to that particular hormone. That location is called a receptor site. The hormones and neurotransmitters "dock" into the receptors, signaling the cell to action. This is a critical step in the regulatory function of the body.

Receptors are easily damaged by inflammation and free radicals, thus interrupting proper regulation of the body. There are multiple steps in this sequence that can become damaged and cause problems. A brief description of these steps is as follows:

1. Secretion of the hormone, usually from a gland or organ
2. Transport of the hormone in the bloodstream
3. Docking of the hormone into receptors
4. Activation of function inside the cell

If one could count the receptors in the body, the total number would be staggering. There are receptors for movement and position in space (mechanoreceptors). There are receptors for vision, hearing, touch, taste, and smell. There are receptors for hormones and neurotransmitters. Even blood pressure and chemicals have receptors. Every action in our bodies is initiated by receptors responding to information carried by hormones and chemicals.

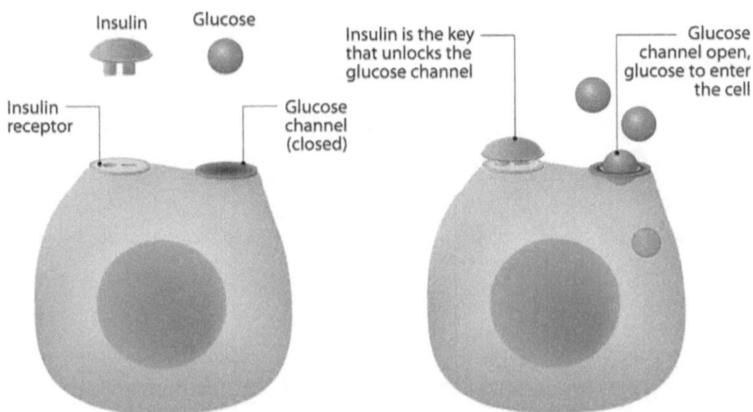

Insulin Receptor© Designua | Dreamstime.com

The image above is an illustration of a receptor for insulin. Hormones dock into receptors, which opens up the cell, allowing glucose to pass into the cell. Think of the receptor as a boat dock. The boat parks in the dock and the passengers depart, carrying goods and information. If the boat is too big—i.e., the receptor is damaged—it will not fit in the dock and the passengers cannot depart and deliver their goods.

Serotonin is another wonderful example of a neurotransmitter that docks in to a receptor. You may be familiar with serotonin because of its well documented roll in depression. It was once believed that most, if not all, serotonin receptors were located in the brain. Further research has revealed that the gut lining contains 95 percent of the serotonin receptors in the entire body.[2] The gut communicates with the brain and the brain communicates with the gut. Inflammation disrupts this vital communication by damaging the lining of the gut and killing the beneficial bacteria (flora) that produce serotonin in the first place. Overcoming depression most certainly involves restoring the health of the gut lining and replenishing the flora that colonize within the gut.

The Enemy for all Receptors

The shape of each receptor and the hormones which dock there is vitally important. If the receptors and hormones have been damaged from inflammation and poor diet, the shape of the receptors is altered. The signaling process cannot take place as it was designed. (Type 2 diabetes is called "insulin resistance" because the receptors for insulin become damaged, which keeps the cell from responding to insulin.) Toxins are a major player in the inflammatory process that alters receptor function.

Health Tip: Just as the body responds to hormones, it also responds to synthetic chemicals and toxins.

The Toxic Effect on Receptors

BPA (Bisphenyl A) is one of many examples of a potent toxic chemical. BPA is commonly used in flexible plastics. It is also used on the inner lining of commercial canned goods.

The reason BPA is so destructive is that it occupies receptors designed for other hormones. By occupying these receptors, BPA mimics the effects of estrogens in females and males and it blocks insulin receptors. For the female, BPA causes overstimulation of the ovaries with a nasty form of estrogen that causes menstrual irregularities, insulin resistance, overdevelopment of breast tissue, and cancer of the breast and uterus. In males, BPA causes shrinking of the testicles, feminization of the male body, and prostate cancer.

BPA disrupts insulin and blood sugar handling as well. This and other chemicals covered in chapter 8 and 9 are known as endocrine (hormone) disruptors that have devastating effects on the body.

Cholesterol, Omega-3s, and Statin Drugs: How They Tie Together

Previously I wrote about general statistics related to the use of statin drugs, commonly prescribed to lower cholesterol. What seems harmless can actually create major problems for the body. Since this is a chapter on the important role of cell membranes and lipids, this is a perfect time to include some details behind the statements I made in chapter two because statin drugs directly affect the lipid balance in the body.

First, understand that cholesterol is a lipid that is vital to the health of the body. In addition to dietary sources, cholesterol is manufactured by the liver. The body uses cholesterol to produce a variety of other hormones, such as vitamin D, testosterone, and estrogen, as well as neurotransmitters (thirty-two, to be exact). Production of these hormones is dependent upon proper cholesterol levels. The brain and nervous system depend on cholesterol for healthy regeneration. This is the key point to understand. Statin drugs enter the picture because they lower cholesterol in the blood under the pretense of two basic assumptions: (1) diets high in cholesterol create high cholesterol levels in the blood, and (2) high blood cholesterol causes the arteries to clog up, causing heart disease.

In my opinion, and the opinion of many other researchers, the theory linking cholesterol to heart disease should be updated to more appropriately match the information in the current scientific literature. To cling to outdated theory helps no one and stands in the way of truly helping mankind. It has been proven that cholesterol is just an innocent bystander in the onset and progression of heart disease. Inflammation is the key player in the onset of heart disease. As cholesterol circulates in the blood, two things happen if the person is inflamed: (1) the inflammation damages (oxidizes) the cholesterol, which makes it more prone to adhere to artery walls, and (2) the inflammation damages the lining of the artery, which readily forms plaque that sticks to the walls of the artery. Studies have shown that many people who have heart disease and suffer from heart attacks have high levels of the inflammatory chemical C-reactive protein, an inflammation marker, in their blood. And a large percentage of heart disease patients do not have high cholesterol at all. When the synthesis of cholesterol is blocked, driving cholesterol to unsafe low levels, there are serious consequences to overall health and well-being.

Anything that decreases cholesterol to unsafe levels, whether it is the inability of the liver to produce its own cholesterol (liver disease) or a statin drug given to lower cholesterol, could cause a slow but progressive decay (atrophy) of the brain and the nerves. This is commonly what is seen in Alzheimer's disease. As the brain shrinks, cognitive function slowly declines. Statin drugs are not the only cause of Alzheimer's disease (AD), but they are definitely a contributing factor. It is interesting to note that new cases of Alzheimer's have doubled since 1982, the year statins were introduced. New cases of AD are expected to rise 44 percent by the year 2025.[3] At our present rate, that rise would parallel the rise in statin use.

Statins are also known to deplete a vital antioxidant from the body called CoQ10. CoQ10 happens to be heart protective, so depleting it increases the risk of a heart attack. If you are taking a statin drug, it would be wise to take supplemental CoQ10 to offset the loss initiated by consumption of the statin. In addition, research shows that statin drugs suppress a vital chemical in the blood called Nuclear Factor Kappa B, which helps the body fight infection and form an immune response against cancer cells.[4] Even by 2004 deaths from cancer due to long term statin therapy was being reported in the literature, leading some researchers to conclude that the risk of long term statin use outweighs the benefits.

So where is the good news in all of this? The good news is that studies clearly show the benefits of fish oil in the cholesterol debate. This provides consumers with a viable option to statin drugs, which addresses the core issue of heart disease: inflammation. One comparative study between statin drugs and omega-3 oils (from fish oil) came to an interesting conclusion.[5] In the study, omega-3 oils were compared to statin drugs in clinical effectiveness for lowering cholesterol *and* for lowering the risk of death from a heart attack. Decreasing the risk of heart attack and stroke is the sole reason for statins. The question is in the safety of their use.

So how did the study conclude?

Overall, omega-3s decreased cholesterol levels by an average of 2 percent, compared to 20 percent for statin drugs. But this is where it gets interesting:

Omega-3s showed a 44 percent greater reduction in deaths from heart attacks than statins. Plus, omega-3s showed a 32 percent greater reduction in deaths from other causes, such as blood clots and inflammatory diseases.

Researchers concluded that omega-3s are more effective at preventing death from heart attacks and other causes because:

- They are anti-inflammatory.
- They thin the blood and reduce clotting.
- They stabilize heart rhythm.
- They help cell membranes stay fluid.
- They improve the body's response to hormones.

Many research studies have supported that fish oil is safe even in high doses as long as it is purified from contaminants and coupled with a rich supply of antioxidants.[6] This is encouraging because many of these studies on fish oil have been performed using doses as high as ten grams. The results are promising and show positive responses in cases of brain disorders, chronic pain, and heart disease.[7, 8]

The research also suggests that there are safer ways to address the root cause of heart disease than through the use of statins. Since *inflammation* is the source of arterial disease, it would make sense to address the inflammatory response first.

Is it ever appropriate to take a statin drug? Only you and your doctor can ultimately make that decision. If your cholesterol and triglycerides are significantly elevated, yes, it may be appropriate to take a statin drug for a short period of time—at least until diet and exercise modifications can be made. It is interesting to note that statin drugs do have a mild anti-inflammatory component, which accounts for their reduction of heart attacks in the literature. The marginal effectiveness of statin drugs at decreasing heart attacks was never about lowering cholesterol. Some individuals even have a higher genetic predisposition for elevated cholesterol levels, which again makes it risky to force the body to lower cholesterol levels.

Additional natural alternatives include red rice yeast and policosanol. These are natural compounds that have been shown to reduce cholesterol. These compounds are safe in small doses but should only be taken under a physician's supervision because of the likelihood of other factors that may be contributing to high cholesterol, such as insulin resistance (covered in chapter six).

Blood Tests for Inflammation Markers

It is common for physicians to order blood tests to determine their patients' cholesterol levels. The question is not in the value of testing cholesterol and other blood fats (lipids); the question is in the interpretation of the tests. Elevated blood lipids are a sign of blood sugar handling issues and liver dysfunction, especially seen in type 2 diabetes. Lowering cholesterol does not address this or other potential issues.

It is equally important to order blood tests to determine the patient's inflammation levels in addition to blood lipids. Inflammation markers are a much greater indicator of whether or not you are at risk for a heart attack or stroke. These are the tests you can request from your doctor when having a routine physical examination:

1. C-reactive protein, homocysteine, insulin, and VLDL blood tests. The first three are considered markers of inflammation. Inflammation plays a key role in the onset of heart disease as concluded by a 2002 study:[9]

- The study, published in the *New England Journal of Medicine* cited elevated C-reactive protein as the strongest predictor for heart attack and stroke. Medical journals use the word predictor to literally mean an elevated test predicts the person will have a heart attack if the cause of the inflammation is not addressed. If used correctly, this preventive blood test is a sign that lifestyle changes are needed to avoid future problems. Because C-reactive protein is a marker of inflammation, it is also a predictor of other vascular problems, such as the lung disorder COPD.[10] This is even more evidence that inflammation is at the root of some serious chronic diseases.
- VLDL are the small particles of cholesterol that stick to artery walls. Testing C-reactive protein and VLDL together is better than either marker tested individually.[11]
- Homocysteine is a marker for inflammation but also a marker for the MTHFR genetic defect that impairs methylation (detoxification). Prolonged impaired methylation is associated with heart disease and higher incidence of stroke. Elevated homocysteine can be effectively managed with supplemental use of methylated folic acid, methylated vitamin B-12, vitamin B6, and SAMe.[12] SAMe is an abbreviation for S-Adenosyl Methionine, one of the most powerful compounds that assists in turning on the methylation process, also discussed in chapter 9.
- Insulin is a necessary hormone that regulates blood sugar. Elevated insulin levels are a strong indicator of insulin resistance seen in type 2 diabetes, discussed in chapter 6.[13,14] Insulin is highly inflammatory because it drives the conversion of Arachidonic acid to PGE2.

Note: Be aware that your insurance company may deny payment for these tests under the "not medically necessary" category. You may have to pay for these tests out of pocket.

If your doctor is resistant, ask him or her to agree to a time frame in which you will work to get your levels under control through diet and exercise. Six months is a reasonable request before retesting your levels again. Most doctors will be willing to work with you. Don't make this request if you're not willing to put in the work to help yourself. Follow an anti-inflammatory diet of vegetables; fruit; lean protein, such as chicken and fish; and nuts and seeds, such as almonds, cashews, pistachios, and sunflower seeds. Stay well hydrated with plenty of water, and avoid sugar and soda. Take plenty of antioxidants, fish oil, vitamin D, and probiotics for gut health. Probiotics are beneficial bacteria that live in the intestines, keeping the environment in the intestines healthy. Among their many attributes, probiotics aid in proper digestion and elimination, but also assist in manufacture of key vitamins in the intestinal tract.

If these recommendations still do not produce the desired results, consider consulting a chiropractor, naturopath, or nutritionist who has knowledge of the things we've discussed.

2. Another predictive blood test is the AA/EPA ratio. AA, of course, is Arachidonic acid, the inflammation-producing bad fat. EPA is the major anti-inflammatory omega-3 fat.

The majority of blood tests reveal problems *after* they occur. The preventive value of most blood tests is diminished somewhat by the fact that problems often show up in the blood long after the actual problem began. The AA/EPA ratio is one of the few blood tests predictive of future problems long *before* they occur, thus giving the person time to make the necessary lifestyle changes to prevent the onset of disease.

This test is a ratio just like other blood lipid tests. The AA/EPA ratio tells the amount of inflammatory bad fats versus anti-inflammatory good fats in the blood. Anything over 10:1 is a strong predictor of degenerative disease and cancer. It is not an indicator that you have cancer; it is an indicator that you are headed for cancer or degenerative disease if you continue down the same path. A high AA/EPA ratio occurs from overconsumption of bad fats and under consumption of quality omega-3 fats.[15, 16]

In western cultures, as the consumption of bad fats from vegetable oils has exploded, so has the decline in consumption of quality omega-3 fats. This is not a fair trade, as this shift in fat consumption is a major factor in the increased rates of cancer and chronic illness in western cultures. This increase in bad fats parallels the rise of corn and soy in the western diet. One tablespoon of corn oil contains 7.3 grams of inflammatory omega-6 fats, and one tablespoon of soybean oil contains 6.9 grams of inflammatory omega-6 fats. One large serving of french fries contains as much as 37 grams of inflammation-inducing fat. This should provide some perspective on how much of these oils most Americans consume.

Even animal feed has not escaped this trend, as corn and soy have become a staple feed for cows, hogs, and poultry. Commercial farmers have been known to add used vegetable oil from fast-food restaurants to feed for their cattle. They get fat in a hurry but they become unhealthy cows.

As I was reading the literature for this section, I found it interesting that average AA/EPA ratios have exploded from 2:1 (where they should be) in the early 1900s to nearly 25:1 today (where they shouldn't be). Our diets have changed significantly and it shows in the AA/EPA ratios of each generation. If 10:1 or above is in the danger zone and the average American is 25:1, this is not good news; it is more evidence that our diets are impacting our health in everything from chronic pain to chronic illness.[17] Studies have shown that people suffering from schizophrenia have AA/EPA ratios as high as 70:1. This alone suggests there is a strong dietary connection to schizophrenia and other depressive disorders.

Again the AA/EPA ratio is not a test that shows pathological diseases. It is an early predictor for changes in inflammatory fats in the blood that lead to pathological changes, such as cancer. These changes show up long before the actual signs of any disease. Even if you have not been diagnosed with cancer, if you are in this range, you are headed for trouble. It is a preventive blood test. I encourage you to have and your loved ones and yourself tested.

Beyond the Cell

In concluding this chapter, I feel it is important to go deeper, beyond the cell, to the level of subatomic particles because this is where health and disease originate. This is one of the fascinating mysteries that bridge the gap between science and theology. As I said at the beginning of this chapter, on a quantum level the cell is essentially a cluster of atoms that are formed together in a cohesive unit. If we look at a cell through a high-powered electron microscope, we will see clusters of atoms with electrons spinning around the nucleus. The forces that hold the atoms together and keep the electrons moving are invisible, but we know they exist through the laws of quantum physics. Scientists literally call these strong and weak forces. Here's where it gets interesting.

We know the cells of different organs have different tissue types, but what is it that makes them different when they all have similar atoms? The atoms that make up the healthy cell are exactly the same as the diseased cell. I call it grand design. Here's why.

A low-powered microscope shows us clear and visible differences in structure and function of healthy cells and diseased cells. If we magnify a healthy cell and a cancer cell down to their smallest components, we will see subatomic particles called quarks and leptons. These subatomic particles are so small, they have no measurable shape or mass. Quarks are in a constant state of motion. They spin around an axis, much like the earth. Unlike the earth, quarks can randomly change the direction in which they spin. The fact that they have no mass and no shape means the only thing left when you reach the level of a quark is energy. Not just any energy, this energy is coherent, meaning it's organized. It has an intelligence that governs the cell, including the DNA.

If we looked at the quarks of these two specimens, they would appear exactly the same. The visible difference at the cellular level disappears when we reach the quantum level. The only true difference is the vibrational resonance of each respective cell. The difference in resonance could be due to the diseased cell gaining or losing electrons, thus changing the rate in which the electrons spin around the nucleus. This is the definition of free-radical-induced inflammation. My understanding of quantum physics leads me to believe that quarks are the building block of all matter, including thought itself. And, the change in the vibration of electrons and quarks alters the structure and function of the cells. This is Gods grand design at its finest!

Author Wayne Dyer had some keen insight when he made the observation that quantum theory and theology are tied together in this verse from scripture, which I found absolutely brilliant:

> Through faith we understand that the worlds were framed by the word of God, so that things which are seen were not made of things which do appear. Hebrews 11:3 (KJV)

Dr. Dyer was translating the words eloquently penned by the Apostle Paul to mean, particles (cells) don't create themselves. There has to be an infusion of spirit (God) to have physical form of any sort, whether it's a healthy cell, a cancer cell, or any other living being. Where does spirit come from? Again referring to scripture:

> And the Lord God formed man of the dust of the ground, and breathed into his nostrils the breath of life; and man became a living soul. Genesis 2:7 (KJV)

If the difference between two cells truly lies in the resonance of each individual cell, there must be an interruption of spirit that manifests in a cell expressing disease. Therefore, healing of any disease has to be a result of changing the resonance of the diseased tissue. In theological terms, becoming one with the spirit that created us literally changes us from the inside out. This is the scientific explanation of how prayer heals our body. We become one with that which created us, and thus, the miracle of healing occurs.

Tying It All Together

Toxins create free radicals. Free radicals promote inflammation. Inflammation changes the resonance at the atomic level, which filters back up the chain through the cells, organs, and tissues. The tissues express the change in resonance as disease. That which is seen did not come from that which appears.

Our eyes play tricks on us. The things we see are only a fraction of what appears in front of us. The things we don't see with our eyes have tremendous influence over our bodies. The food we eat and the thoughts that fill our heads have a major influence on the atoms and quarks deep within our cells. This concept stretches the limits of the imagination, but it truly uncovers universal truths that affect all of us.

If someone asks you how your quarks are doing, you can say that they're vibrating nicely, thank you.

CHAPTER 6

The Diabetes Epidemic

Obesity rates have risen dramatically over the last twenty years; make that exploded. It is now estimated that nearly 50 percent of Americans are considered obese. That is nearly 160 million people based on current population estimates. Even more alarming, it is estimated that nearly 70 percent of Americans suffer from type 2 diabetes. The technical term for type 2 diabetes is "insulin resistance," but it is also referred to as "metabolic syndrome." They mean the same thing. Type 2 diabetics produce insulin, sometimes in massive amounts, but the insulin cannot do its job of getting sugar inside the cell because the insulin receptors have been damaged or the cell membranes are damaged.

Insulin is knocking on the door, but the cell is not listening.

The body's response is to produce more insulin in an attempt to lower blood sugar. This is called reactive hypoglycemia, which can produce sudden drops in blood sugar in the early stages of the disease, causing extreme fatigue and a jittery feeling in the limbs.

There are some key factors to know about insulin:

1. It promotes inflammation (PGE 2).
2. It signals the conversion of sugar (glucose) into cholesterol (fat).
3. It stimulates the autonomic nervous system.

Insulin is necessary for health, but *excess* insulin is very disruptive. This is why monitoring insulin levels in the blood is so important.[1] Insulin is so important that a key textbook from the American Academy of Pain Management, 2006, seventh edition, says in chapter five: "For effective, long term pain management, inflammatory compounds called eicosanoids (PGE2) should be lowered through dietary changes (increasing omega 3 fats) and by *controlling insulin levels* through reduction of refined carbohydrates.[2] They could've easily stated, for long term prevention of cancer or any disease, bad fats, refined carbohydrates and insulin must be decreased, good fats must be increased.

I can assure you I'm not making this stuff up. From everything I have read, the root cause of disease, including diabetes, is inflammation from free radicals and immune system overstimulation.[3,4]

The Little Engines in Your Cells: Mitochondria

In chapter 5, I mentioned the two key primary parts of the cells that are damaged from inflammation are the outer cell membrane and the mitochondria. Now it is time for us to understand the mitochondria, which are considered to be the powerhouse of the cell because they produce the fuel needed to power the rest of the body. This fuel is called ATP (adenosine triphosphate). Mitochondria are the only cell components that produce ATP, so mitochondrial health is critically important to having a healthy body.

There is one more critical link in the chain for proper energy production in the cells. Mitochondria require starches and fats in the diet and healthy liver function to produce ATP. Starches must be converted to glucose before they can be used to make ATP. This conversion is done exclusively in the liver. If the liver is not functioning correctly due to toxic overload from poor food choices, prescription drugs, or other factors, this conversion process may be hindered. A balanced diet naturally contains the nutrients and enzymes necessary to make this conversion. I'll cover what a balanced diet looks like in chapter ten. For now, just know that ATP production is dependent on the *quality* and *quantity* of starches and fats in the diet.

ATP production occurs in the mitochondria and free radicals cause damage to the energy production inside the cells of the pancreas. Sugar (glucose) cannot be metabolized without ATP. Do you see a problem here? Yes, the energy supply to the cells is compromised. For clarification, this is not referencing processed sugar you buy in the store. Sugar (glucose) is required for healthy energy production. However, the liver must manufacture glucose before it can be utilized. And, the liver and kidneys are responsible for breaking down toxins so they can be excreted from the body. Prolonged ingestion of toxins and chemicals from poor dietary habits will add an extra burden on the liver, which can hinder the conversion of starches to glucose. Toxins can be from many sources—preservatives/additives in processed food, excess consumption of refined carbohydrates and bad fats, or environmental toxins. This is one of several causes of high blood sugar because the liver becomes overloaded, which hinders the proper regulation of blood sugar, and ultimately ATP production suffers. Without ATP production, many diseases, including diabetes and Alzheimer's, are considered to be the end result.

Prolonged excess insulin (type 2 diabetes) progresses to where the pancreas loses the ability to produce insulin. Eventually the person becomes a type 1 diabetic (where not enough insulin is produced). What is happening here is the pancreas is becoming overstimulated while, at the same time, being damaged by inflammation. Organs can become depleted and exhausted just like muscles. The problem is once organs become fatigued and damaged, the condition is difficult to reverse.

In clinical practice I have seen type 2 diabetics with normal blood sugar but massively high insulin levels, indicating insulin resistance. Physicians would do their patients a huge favor if they checked insulin levels along with blood sugar on routine blood checks. This is not routine practice for endocrinologists for various reasons, one being insurance does not pay for the test so it would be an out-of-pocket expense for the patient. Remember, blood sugar can be normal even when insulin is critically high. This is an indicator of distress in the body's sugar-handling and high inflammation levels. Since excessive insulin drives inflammation (PGE2), patients with insulin resistance will likely have fatigue, joint pain, and cloudy thinking, even memory problems. Left unchecked it spirals into a cancerous process.

Health Tip: Excessive insulin is pro-inflammatory and promotes tumor growth. Insist on having your insulin levels checked when you have blood tests done.

In summary: We know that diabetes is caused by the inability to produce ATP energy due to damage in the mitochondria of the pancreas and other cells of the body (important point). Think about it. Glucose and fat are the primary fuel for mitochondria inside the cell. It takes ATP to move glucose and fat into the cell; plus it takes more ATP to convert the glucose and fat to usable forms to power the mitochondria. No ATP means no fuel for the cells. If glucose cannot get into the cell and the engine that runs the cell has no fuel, the energy source for all body parts is compromised, especially the brain. The brain has the highest demand for fuel and oxygen of any organ.

By the way, the most critical organ that runs nearly exclusively from glucose is … *the brain*! No ATP production means the brain is starved for fuel. Friends, this is a bad deal for the body! Since the brain is composed of mostly fat, it is especially susceptible to damage from free radicals. This damage can quickly erode cognitive function.

Current research indicates that people who have Alzheimer's disease have lost the ability to produce ATP energy in their brain. In fact, many researchers are now calling Alzheimer's disease "diabetes of the brain."[5] Some of the latest pharmaceutical drugs for Alzheimer's disease are geared toward getting the brain to absorb sugar again, thereby producing ATP energy and helping the brain do its job. However, one of the most effective non-pharmaceutical alternatives for producing ATP energy in the body is consuming coconut oil. Coconut oil is composed of a specific type of fat called medium chain triglycerides. When a person consumes medium chain triglycerides, it completely bypasses the need for glucose inside the cells to produce ATP by producing ketones.

Ketones are an alternative energy source for the mitochondria, similar in comparison to high vs. low octane gasoline in your car. The high octane fuel produces more power from the engine. The ketones are easily absorbed into the bloodstream and into the cells, producing larger amounts of ATP than glucose. This is the reason coconut oil is promoted as an effective weight-loss supplement because it helps the body utilize insulin more effectively, which stimulates weight loss.

Ketones are also produced from reducing refined carbohydrates and by raising quality proteins and fats in the diet. This type of diet maintains a small amount of ketones in the blood stream, which has shown tremendous benefit in shrinking malignant tumors. Why? Because most cancer cells use glucose for fuel which means the cancer cells have no fuel source.

As a reminder, all ATP energy is produced in the mitochondria, within the cells. What is the most common source of damage to mitochondria? You guessed it, *free radicals*!

Damaged mitochondria not only cannot produce ATP energy, but they also dump free radicals inside the cell, causing further damage.[6,7] Can you see a vicious cycle here? And the majority of this damage begins with dietary habits and stressful thinking, which induces PGE2 and free radical production. How powerful is that?

Understanding Digestion: It's Influence on Blood Sugar

The sequence of digestion goes something like this: John stops at Sonic for lunch. He orders a burger, fries, and a milk shake. The protein, carbohydrates, and fat from the meal have to be digested and absorbed into the bloodstream. First they must be broken down into smaller particles. To simplify, let's pick on the carbohydrates in the bun. The carbs must be broken down to sugar (glucose), which enters the bloodstream with the help of ATP. The sugar must now enter the cell, also with the help of ATP. If the cell is working correctly, insulin from the pancreas docks into the insulin receptors on the outer cell membranes, allowing the sugar to pass through to the inside of the cell. If the insulin receptors are damaged, blood sugar rises excessively; this signals the pancreas to produce more insulin. Again, this is what happens in type two diabetes and is the reason it is called "insulin resistance."

Sugar in the blood cannot pass through the cell membrane because the insulin receptors are damaged, the cell membrane is damaged, or both. Insulin continues to spike higher in an effort to open up the cell. Insulin promotes storage of carbohydrates as fat. Insulin also promotes inflammation, so the longer this process continues, the faster the person becomes overweight and experiences degenerative disease.

The entire goal of digestion is to produce ATP energy to fuel the body's production of new cells and to protect the cells from damage. ATP is used in each step of the digestion process, from digestion of carbs, fats, and proteins into smaller components to moving the smaller components into the bloodstream. It takes even more ATP to move the smaller digested particles into the cells before the nutrients can fuel the mitochondria to produce ATP.

Once inside the bloodstream, the body must decide where the digested material should go. This starts with the chewing process and continues through the stomach and intestines. As the food is mixed with saliva, the proteins, carbohydrates, and fats are "tagged" by enzymes in the saliva. This tagging process assures that the right nutrients go to the right places.

This is a major step in the digestion process that is rendered inefficient by eating too quickly or eating while stressed. This is a good reason to eat slowly and chew your food thoroughly.

Once inside the cell, the mitochondria use sugar (glucose) to produce energy. If the mitochondria are damaged, energy production falters. Inflammation is the primary cause of damage to the cell membrane and the mitochondria. Let's review that process again. Remember, a free radical is essentially an unpaired electron that circulates in the body and damages anything it comes in contact with, especially cell membranes and mitochondria. Damaged mitochondria do not produce adequate amounts of energy (ATP). Furthermore, damaged mitochondria produce more free radicals.

Free-radical damage is often called "oxidative stress." Even though any tissue in the body can undergo oxidative stress, brain and nerve tissue are especially susceptible to damage from free radicals because of their high fat content. The tissue that has been damaged by free radicals now becomes a source of inflammation. Again, inflammation has been linked to nearly every form of degenerative disease, including Parkinson's, Alzheimer's, multiple sclerosis, metabolic syndrome, and many more.

Have you ever wondered why some people look older or younger than they are? It is now believed that exposure to free radicals is what accelerates the aging process, so those who look older than their age are suffering from advanced free-radical damage while those who look younger have protected themselves from free-radical damage.

Other Factors on the Diabetes Epidemic

The lack of physical activity in the younger generation is becoming an ever-increasing problem. Thirty years ago, kids could be found running, jumping, and playing outside in the sunshine. There was meaningful human interaction every day. Now, with the age of computers and cell phones, many children communicate almost exclusively through text messages and social media.

Beyond the lack of physical activity, the constant stimulation from television, computers, and cell phones can have an over stimulating effect on the brain. Studies show that children who frequently watch television in the first three years of life have a dramatically increased risk of developing attention deficit disorder by the time they reach the age of seven. Studies have also shown a link between television viewing in the early years of life and a higher incidence of juvenile diabetes by the age of seven. [8]

Lack of physical activity combined with the tendency to over consume common junk foods while watching television is only the beginning. The overstimulation of the dopamine centers of the brain at an early age is an even bigger issue. The brain becomes addicted to violent acts seen on TV and in movies, desensitizing the child to violence, explosions, and the like. A slow disconnect happens in the child's awareness of right and wrong.[9]

CHAPTER 7

Dietary Toxins

> There is now no question that accumulated toxins are behind nearly every disease, symptom, injury and malfunction of the body.
>
> —Sherry Rogers, MD
> *Detoxify or Die*

Over the past fifty years we have seen a remarkable shift in our food supply. This transition to processed food began in the 1950s and continues to this day. Quick and convenient has become the priority for most households in the form of prepared, packaged foods and drive-through value meals. They are such a part of our culture that it's hard to escape the effects of processed food and synthetic chemicals, even for families who still prepare their meals from scratch. Our culture caters to quick and convenient foods. The ingredients used in packaged foods often have little food value left by the time they reach your dinner plate. And packaged foods are filled with synthetic chemicals, dyes, and preservatives that the body must detoxify (remove) as they are consumed.

Detoxification is a vital process that keeps the body operating correctly by converting toxic chemicals into harmless substances that can be excreted through the kidneys or the liver. Both use specific methods to eliminate toxins. These are called detoxification pathways. If these pathways do not operate efficiently, the toxins build up in the body and cause a host of problems. This is a key part of understanding detoxification. It takes an energy source (fuel) inside the cells to drive detoxification, but this energy source must be manufactured. The fuel is called adenosine triphosphate

(ATP); the same ATP discussed in the previous chapter. But there is one more critical step we can't forget. Glucose (sugar) and fat from the diet are the fuel that turns the engines that manufacture ATP.

Unfortunately, as more chemicals are consumed, the more overloaded the detoxification pathways become in the liver and kidneys, making it difficult for toxins to be eliminated correctly. The inevitable result of faulty detoxification is damage to internal components of the cells. The immune system and the hormonal system can become compromised. Some toxins are so potent they even damage the DNA inside the cells. (Remember, DNA contains the genetic code that helps your body reproduce itself.) The end result is a body with cells that cannot eliminate toxins *and* cannot reproduce healthy cells correctly. That is a lethal combination. Remember, the body is in a continual state of breakdown and repair. The lining of the gut and many other vital organs are replaced every day with new, healthy cells.

We often take for granted that the things we eat today will serve as the fuel that rebuilds our bodies tomorrow. Remind yourself of that important fact and choose your food wisely. This is a key piece of the puzzle that causes disease. Don't allow yourself to be one of the millions of people who continually sow the wrong seeds and end up reaping a horrible disease as a result of those choices. Believe me, over the years in my clinical practice I have heard the story so many times: "I was healthy until I was forty and then the floodgates opened." Now we see the reasons why. The body is very resilient when it has the proper fuel and protective antioxidants. Never forget that.

Toxins in the Diet: What and Where?

Toxins have become commonplace in the standard American diet, so common that it becomes a bit frustrating to find foods without chemicals. But it helps to know the basics of where they come from and how to spot them on labels.

I love to cook steak and chicken on the grill. It's one of my favorite things to do on a warm summer evening. I was pretty disappointed when I learned that cooking meats on the grill generates a host of cancer-causing chemicals as a byproduct of the cooking process. Cooking food, especially at high temperatures, creates chemicals that can produce free radicals and inflammation. One such chemical that has received more attention from scientists in recent years is a toxic byproduct called an AGE (advanced glycation end product). The word *glyco* means sugar (glucose). If sugar becomes glycated, it means the sugar is combined with another substance, usually a protein. This information gets a little complicated so I'll try to simplify it as much as possible.

There are two types of AGE's: those that form outside the body (external), usually through cooking of food, and those that form inside the body (internal) through inflammation.

In summary, an external AGE is formed when starches and proteins within the food you're cooking combine under heat to form a toxic byproduct. Not all AGEs are bad; many occur naturally in small amounts in different types of food. The naturally occurring form has little effect on the body. Toxic AGEs are a different story. The highest amount of *toxic* AGEs come from cooking animal proteins, such as red meat and poultry, and cooking starchy foods in fat or oil, such as french fries, potato chips, crackers, or cookies. I think I just described a large part of the foods we love to eat.

How the food is cooked is a major player in the *amount* and *potency* of the toxic byproducts. The cooking process, especially grilling, broiling, roasting, searing, and frying, accelerates new AGE formation because the cooking is done under high heat. Unfortunately this is the toxic stuff. The good news is boiling and cooking at lower temperatures can reduce toxic AGE formation. Many of the grilling books I have read recommend grilling meats on a high temperature setting over four hundred degrees. Just turn your heat down to three hundred and increase your cooking time, and you can decrease AGE formation. Another helpful tip is to marinade meats in an acidic solution, such as lemon juice or vinegar, for an hour prior to cooking. Marinating has been shown to reduce toxic AGE formation by nearly 50 percent.[1]

Vegetables, fruits, non-GMO whole grains, and low-fat dairy products like cottage cheese have the lowest amount of AGEs of all foods.

Toxic AGEs are bad for the body. Once the starches and proteins are chemically altered from cooking, they generate inflammation in the bloodstream. Inflammation in the bloodstream creates more AGEs. It's a vicious cycle.

Internal AGEs are created when proteins in the blood (like hemoglobin from red blood cells) combine with sugar, forming a substance called glycated hemoglobin. The hemoglobin is literally attaching itself to sugar molecules in the blood stream. Once hemoglobin becomes glycated, the red blood cells carrying the hemoglobin become less efficient at carrying oxygen, which is a bad deal for the body. In fact, glycated hemoglobin leads to reduced oxygen delivery to the tissues, which can produce a specific type of free radical called the *oxygen free radical.* Mitochondria require oxygen to produce ATP. Decreased oxygen supply (hypoxia) creates these free radicals which damages tissue, especially the lungs where the red blood cells pick up more oxygen.

Have you noticed an increase in the number of elderly who carry portable oxygen tanks? Many can't survive without them. Ever wonder why this is happening? Some are lifelong smokers, which makes sense. However, many oxygen users have never smoked in their life. Prolonged exposure to inflammatory free radicals damages the entire chain of oxygen delivery from the red blood cells to the lungs. Dietary AGE's are a major factor in many lung diseases.

Again, the literature is pretty clear that inflammatory conditions accelerate formation of this type of internal AGE, called glycated hemoglobin.[2, 3, 4] High levels of glycated hemoglobin can have severe consequences because of reduced oxygen capacity, which decreases oxygen delivery to the tissues. Reducing the red blood cells' capacity for oxygen produces even more inflammation (oxygen free radicals) through a condition called hypoxia. In addition, waste products that are normally transported out of the body are not eliminated efficiently either. Be aware that free radicals, overstimulation of the immune system, and the inability to remove toxic waste will accelerate the production of cancer and degenerative disease. This was discussed in previous chapters. We're just seeing the effects of the inflammation in the blood stream.

Progress to Deeper Understanding of the Body

The significance of AGEs in the blood has only recently been understood. The blood test that measures glycated hemoglobin is called hemoglobin A1c (HA1c).[5] This can be a predictor for diabetes but is also a predictor of cancer if left unchecked. I say "can be" because a diet high in antioxidants protects red blood cells from destruction (hemolysis), so as red blood cells live longer, this will artificially elevate HA1c to a certain degree. The person reading the test needs to take this into consideration and not just assume diabetes is involved.

Medical guidelines indicate that a normal HA1c is 5.7 or below. A small amount of glycated hemoglobin is considered normal. Here's the problem: For every 1 percent elevation in A1c, there is an 18 percent elevation in cancer risk. A1c only becomes *elevated* if blood sugar is also elevated. The reason for the higher cancer rate is quite simple: sugar and insulin accelerate malignant tumor formation.[6]

Even in the midst of a potentially destructive process, I still can see the grand design of the body at work. High blood sugar is a potentially life-threatening condition. The body is struggling to maintain a healthy blood sugar. The body senses this, so the red blood cells soak up the extra sugar by attaching themselves to the sugar molecules. The end result, rising glycosylated hemoglobin levels, can still cause problems, but the body is buying time and avoiding an immediate crisis: diabetic coma and possible death from hyperglycemia.

The solution to keeping a low HA1c is a diet with minimal refined carbohydrates, in favor of complex carbohydrates, plenty of vegetables, quality sources of fats, and loads of antioxidants. Hemoglobin A1c is also reduced by cooking food at lower temperatures and increasing cooking times accordingly. There are grill masters who may not like these recommendations. I understand. But I would counter the objections with a reminder that we eat to provide fuel for our bodies and not only for pleasure. Cooking food in the safest way possible is as important as eating and enjoying good-tasting food.

AGEs, Carbs, and Health

Diets high in AGEs are associated with higher rates of heart disease, kidney disease, type 1 and type 2 diabetes, Alzheimer's disease, and even cancer. Sound familiar? These are the chronic diseases I listed in chapter two that we have difficulty controlling.

Excessive forms of refined carbohydrates also have been associated with higher rates of cancer because they form AGEs and stimulate insulin, which are inflammatory and tumorigenic. The reason for this connection has not been well understood until recently. People routinely consume large amounts of refined carbohydrates that also contain large amounts of refined oils. This has historically been adopted as the American diet. Refined carbohydrates cause a prolonged spike in blood sugar (hyperglycemia) and high blood insulin levels. Hyperglycemia initiates cancerous tumor growth (it feeds cancer). Once again we see the destructive effects of PGE2 from chapter two.

Now we know that consuming AGEs enhances the growth of cancerous tumors as well. Here is some proof of that destructive process:

A 2005 study published in the *International Journal of Cancer* concluded that consuming one weekly serving of french fries (AGEs formed from cooking potatoes in oil) before puberty resulted in a 27 percent increase in adult onset breast cancer. An additional 44 percent increase in cancer rate was noted from one daily serving of ground beef when consumed with the french fries. That's a potential 71 percent increase in cancer risk from over consuming burgers and fries. This is the traditional meal of a hamburger and french fries that has been a staple of the American diet since the 1940s. Anyone who knows a teenager knows that one weekly serving is not even close to what teens are consuming today. Some eat fries multiple times a day which raises the risk of breast cancer to 44 percent.[7]

The key point here is that diets *low* in AGEs and refined carbohydrates and *high* in antioxidants and good fats have the *lowest* rates of chronic disease, including cancer.

Another interesting fact to note; the research regarding raw coconut oil points to the oil as a factor in reducing insulin and tumor growth. Coconut oil provides a specific type of fat called medium chain triglycerides that provides ATP energy for the body while starving tumor cells. Most, if not all cancer cells use sugar as a source of fuel. Likewise, cancer cells are starved of their fuel source when medium chain triglycerides are used in the diet.

Everyone should take this seriously. No one is immune from the destructive process caused by AGE's. How do we do that? What seems to be a difficult undertaking is really simpler than it appears, as represented by a study found in a 2011 edition of the *Journal of Nutrition and Metabolism.* The study concluded that "cancer prevention is either in stopping the onset of tumor growth or the sufficient delay of tumor growth so that it remains undetected (insignificant) through the person's lifetime. There is significant evidence that even modest reductions in dietary carbohydrates may influence both of these mechanisms positively." This means don't wait until it's too late to make dietary changes. Start by making small changes, but by all means start those changes now before it's too late.[8]

The sad part about the explosion in cancer and chronic diseases is that it's completely preventable by consuming an abundance of anti-inflammatory foods and antioxidants and lowering the intake of glycosylated foods.

The question is do we just throw up our hands and concede that people are going to overindulge in AGEs no matter what the consequences? Should we just happily treat the cancer cases as they appear? That is essentially what we are doing right now. Or do we educate the consumer (*you*) that cancer will be the likely end result if you choose to eat an overabundance of refined carbohydrates that turn into glycosylated end products in the blood. Which makes the most sense to you?

We have done a poor job of educating consumers on this issue. Just saying, "french fries are bad for you" is not enough to get people's attention. People need to know *why* they are bad and what the consequences are if they choose to consume them on a regular basis. An occasional order of fries is not going to kill you. Prolonged consumption is where the problem lies.

Bread: The Delight of the Fast-Food Industry and Carb Junkies

Most commercial bread and pastries are produced with enriched flour. Look on the label and it literally says "enriched flour." Sometimes it says brominated flour. It sounds harmless, but it's actually quite disruptive to the body. Here's why. Bread is made of wheat. The outer part of the wheat kernel contains most of the nutrition. Using unrefined whole wheat flour adds bulk to the bread, which is somehow a bad thing to bread makers. Bread makers strip the kernel from the wheat using acid and chemicals as it is being processed. In order to add some nutrition back into the bread, the dough is "enriched" with a synthetic soup of "brominated chemicals."

Bromine is a halide mineral, much like chlorine. It has a nasty affinity for iodine receptors. Where are most iodine receptors located? The thyroid, breast, prostate, and brain. Iodine activates normal metabolism in these tissues. As bromine blocks these receptors, the tissues become dysfunctional and cannot produce hormones or carry out normal metabolism efficiently.[9] This is yet another example of how our food is slowly poisoning our population. Brominated flour is not a necessary ingredient for a simple loaf of bread.

Always look for non-enriched flour or whole wheat flour in baked goods or simply buy organic when possible. It may cost more, but the extra cost is worth it to spare your body the effects of brominated flour.

The food industry has been under a greater microscope in recent years, thanks to documentaries like *Food, Inc.* and *Super Size Me*. If you have not seen these documentaries, I would encourage you to do so. They are eye-opening. Brominated chemicals are disruptive and should be avoided, especially if you have thyroid problems or any other hormonal issues. If you don't have hormonal problems, eating brominated baked goods will accelerate your chances of having them.

Toxic Antibiotics

One of the common practices of the commercial poultry industry is to fatten their chickens faster through the use of chemicals. They can produce a full-grown chicken 30 percent faster by exposing the chickens to a bath of antibiotics and arsenic, which are appetite stimulants. Arsenic, by the way, has long been the chemical of choice for rat poison. The chickens become so top heavy that they literally cannot stand up when fully grown. They just topple over.

What are the effects of these chemicals on the human body? You guessed it. Appetite stimulation, along with stimulation of estrogens, overgrowth of female breasts, fibrocystic breasts, ovarian and uterine cysts, and insulin resistance. Higher cancer rates have been noted as well. In males, hormonal issues, such as erectile dysfunction and low sperm count, are the end result.

Don't expect a ban on the use of these chemicals anytime soon. There is too much pressure from lobbyists and special interest groups for that to happen. The only way it will change is for you, the consumer, to become educated on what you are eating and simply stop buying commercial products that were manufactured using synthetic chemicals. Always buy organic when possible or raise your own chickens or find a trusted source that is chemical free.

Harmful Effects of Prescription Antibiotics

For many people, antibiotics have been a lifesaver. There are times when the body loses its capacity to fight infection and antibiotics are needed to assist the immune system in fighting off infection. Still, there is a dark side to antibiotic use that has been documented. Repetitive antibiotic use in young females has been found to be a causative agent in breast cancer later in life. This link has been specially noted for antibiotics used in ear infections and acne. I would guess that few parents are aware of this when they allow their children to be placed on repetitive doses of antibiotics early in life.

It is well known that antibiotics have a strong effect on destroying intestinal flora, suppressing immune system reactions, and increasing inflammation. Any one of these factors can be associated with increased risk of cancer. The cause of these various forms of cancer is thought to be through production of PGE2 from the antibiotic. (Remember him, the number one dietary cancer-causing chemical? Only this time the antibiotic is producing him.) Tetracycline has been specifically noted for increasing PGE2, though all forms of antibiotics could be implicated. Physicians and patients should be aware that repeated exposure to antibiotics is a risk factor for developing breast cancer and find alternatives for repeated infections.[10, 11, 12]

Health Tip: Research has proven that adjustments to the upper cervical spine are effective for ear infections in children.[13]

When treating children with ear infections, my clinical experience has been consistent with the health tip above and the research. Anatomically, the eustachian tubes that connect the inner ear to the mouth are straighter and less coiled in a child than in an adult. This allows bacteria to migrate from the mouth to the ear much easier, creating a higher tendency for ear infections in a child. Children frequently have subluxations (misalignments) in the upper vertebrae of the neck, which lower the child's resistance to infection and can irritate the eustachian tube as well. Most ear infections in children respond quickly to upper cervical (neck) adjustments and low doses of bifidus-factor probiotics, much to the delight of sleepless moms and dads who are often at the end of their rope when they bring their child in for treatment.

Since antibiotics are known to kill friendly bacteria, as well as the unfriendly bacteria, it is necessary to take probiotics after taking antibiotics to reestablish healthy bacteria in the gut. Altered flora in the gut lowers resistance to future infections. This is a major cause of repeated infections, as gut flora becomes more and more depleted from repeated use of antibiotics. Since there is a direct correlation between the gut and the brain, alterations in gut flora early in life have been linked with behavior disorders, such as ADD and autism. This is definitely grounds for being mindful of repeated exposure to antibiotics or other chemicals that alter bacteria balance in the gut.

CHAPTER 8

Environmental Toxins in Everyday Life

Toxic exposure comes from many sources. In the last chapter we looked at toxins generated during the cooking process. In this chapter we will look at toxic exposure from the environment. Some toxins are used as food additives. Some come from various types of pollution. They are all destructive.

Toxins are *very* difficult to eliminate completely because they're in just about everything. But they can be reduced. This should be everyone's goal. It starts with learning what they are and how to avoid them.

Table 4 illustrates some common toxins that are known to cause health problems. You may recognize some of these from food labels.

Table 4: Common Toxins

Food Products		
Toxins	**Where are they?**	**Why are they toxic?**
Enriched (bleached) flour	Endocrine disruptor commonly found in baked goods.	Flour bleached with bromine. It blocks iodine receptors in the thyroid, breast, and prostate.

Grain/corn-fed beef and vegetable oils (safflower, canola, and cottonseed)	Grain/corn-fed beef and baked goods. Omega-6 oils convert to Arachidonic acid (AA) when digested. AA produces a major inflammatory chemical in the body called prostaglandin E2 (PGE2).	Linked with nearly every chronic pain syndrome, arthritis, and cancer. Suppresses the immune system, causes platelets to stick together, and causes brain injury.
Excitotoxins (aspartame and sucralose)	Used as flavor enhancers in food and soft drinks. Sucralose is chlorinated sugar, made by attaching four chlorine molecules to one molecule of sugar.	Linked with over ninety-two diseases of the nervous system and endocrine system, and causes chronic pain syndromes.
	Environmental Toxins	
Toxins	**Where are they?**	**Why are they toxic?**
Phthalates	Chemical in plastics.	Endocrine disruptor, causes shrinking of the testicles and ovaries, causes cancer.
PBDEs (polybrominated diphenyl ether)	Flame retardant found in plastics, paints, solvents, carpet padding, and mattresses.	Endocrine disruptor affecting the thyroid and other hormones. Damages DNA.
PCBs (polychlorinated biphenyls)	Found in plastics and solvents. Does not break down over time. Many of the world's oceans are polluted with PCBs.	Endocrine disruptor that causes many forms of cancer.

Glyphosate	Commercial pesticide still used in the United States but banned in many European countries.	Extremely toxic even in small amounts. Linked to autism, obesity, allergies, inflammatory bowel disorders, depression, cardiovascular disease, cancer, and many more diseases. Damages DNA.
Bisphenol A (BPA)	A synthetic chemical used in the manufacturing of plastics and for lining in commercial canned goods.	Endocrine disruptor that mimics estrogen, causing hormonal imbalances and cancer of the breast and prostate.
Atrazine	The most commonly used pesticide in the United States. Primarily applied to nonorganic corn.	Disrupts the development of ovaries and testicles. Causes cancer in humans.
Parabens	Found in personal hygiene products like shampoo and body wash.	Endocrine system disruptor.
Aluminum	Found in vaccines and some municipal drinking water.	It increases free-radical production and collects in the brain.

Excitotoxins

The term *excitotoxin* was first investigated in 1993 as a possible cause of neurological damage. Dr. Russell Blaylock and others later investigated the topic, and excitotoxins were confirmed to be a common source of damage to the brain and other vital organs. Excitotoxins are chemicals such as monosodium glutamate (MSG) and aspartic acid (aspartame) that are used as flavor enhancers in processed food. These chemicals are extremely toxic to the brain and nerve tissue. They are also identified as a cause of pain syndromes like fibromyalgia, where patients have reported significant pain relief after discontinuing use of products that contain these toxic chemicals. Unfortunately, we still have "experts" who scoff at the notion that excitotoxins exist and deny their powerful effects. They should read the data.

It is important for you, the consumer, to be able to read food labels and spot when excitotoxins are present. Be aware that food labels can be misleading. Hidden sources of monosodium glutamate can be labeled as hydrolyzed vegetable protein or protein isolates. "Natural flavors" on a food label often means the amino acids aspartate and glutamate have been added to the food. These amino acids are highly toxic and should be avoided if you would like to preserve your brain function.[1, 2, 3, 4]

Limiting Toxic Exposure

Limiting toxic exposure cannot be overemphasized. It is a very serious problem. Today, it is estimated that people are exposed to nearly *three thousand* toxic synthetic chemicals every year. Toxic exposure is especially disastrous for the developing fetus and for young children.[5] Chemicals such as lead, mercury, PCBs, arsenic, insecticides, DDT, phthalates, and BPA are some of the common environmental toxins from table four. Be aware that they are everywhere.

The list of disorders these toxins cause should get everyone's attention, especially women who are pregnant and parents of children under six years of age. You'll notice that a common theme among many of these chemicals is they disrupt the hormonal (endocrine) system. This is not a good thing for anyone at any age, but they are especially disruptive to children and developing fetuses because the body depends on hormonal balance for proper development. The detoxification pathways that break down these harmful substances are undeveloped in children and in the fetus, so their effects can be even more significant. Expectant moms should be especially cautious about receiving flu shots during pregnancy because most flu shots still contain the preservative thimerosal, which is 50 percent ethyl mercury. Ethyl mercury is often said to be less toxic than the more potent methyl mercury but this is not completely accurate. For adults this may be the case;

for a child below six years of age the risk increases because of the inability to break down and excrete the mercury. Ethyl mercury readily crosses the placental and the blood brain barrier, making any exposure extremely hazardous.

When discussing toxic exposure to a fetus, it is difficult to measure the origin of the exposure and how much exposure came from the environment. Taking tissue samples directly from a fetus in utero, especially for research purposes, is not always practical. However, researchers have conducted experiments in which random tissue samples were taken from fetal umbilical cords after birth and tested for chemical exposure in the womb. The results of these tests are frightening. More than 232 chemicals have been commonly found in the samples, including BPA, flame retardants and rocket fuel (perchlorate) from frying pans and computer circuit boards. This is exposure in utero. Many of these chemicals cause cancer, insulin resistance and disrupt the hormonal system long before birth.

Nearly three-fourths of the umbilical cords tested contained synthetic musks called galaxolide and tonalide. Synthetic musks are routinely used in commercial soaps, perfumes and colognes. They are known to cause disruption of the body's hormonal system, the sex hormones in particular. These chemicals would certainly damage the sex organs and cause insulin resistance and other hormonal problems in a developing fetus. It's no wonder there is a diabetes epidemic going on across the globe. Children are developing insulin resistance and other hormone imbalances even before they are born.

The data clearly indicates that expectant moms and infants are being contaminated by everyday cosmetics (and many other toxins) during pregnancy. The developing fetus is extremely vulnerable to toxins, primarily because the removal of toxins is regulated by a chemical detoxification process called glutathione methylation, which is undeveloped in infants and children under six years of age.

Toxins From Vaccines

It is estimated that by the time a child reaches six years of age in the United States, he or she has been exposed to over 130 rounds of vaccines. Twenty-six of those are in the first year alone. The United States has the highest vaccine rate in the world. Higher vaccine rates are associated with higher infant mortality. Thirty-three countries that have *fewer* vaccines mandated in the first year of life also have *lower* infant mortality rates than the United States.[6]

The list below includes some of the common additives used in vaccines. This information was accessed from the Centers for Disease Control (CDC) website:

- Suspending fluid (e.g., sterile water, saline, or fluids containing protein)
- Preservatives and stabilizers to help the vaccine remain unchanged (e.g., albumin, phenols, and glycine)
- Adjuvants or enhancers to make the vaccine more effective
- Aluminum gels or salts of aluminum that are added as adjuvants to help the vaccine stimulate a better response. Adjuvants help promote an earlier, more potent response and a more persistent immune response to the vaccine.
- Antibiotics, which are added to some vaccines to prevent the growth of germs (bacteria) during production and storage of the vaccine. No vaccine produced in the United States contains penicillin.
- Egg protein found in influenza and yellow fever vaccines, which are prepared using chicken eggs. Ordinarily, persons who are able to eat eggs or egg products can receive these vaccines safely.
- Formaldehyde, used to inactivate bacterial products for toxoid vaccines (vaccines that use an inactive bacterial toxin to produce immunity). It is also used to kill unwanted viruses and bacteria that might contaminate the vaccine during production. Most formaldehyde is removed from the vaccine before it is packaged.
- Monosodium glutamate (MSG) and 2-phenoxyethanol, which are used as stabilizers in a few vaccines to help the vaccine remain unchanged when it is exposed to heat, light, acidity, or humidity.
- Thimerosal, a mercury-containing preservative added to vials of vaccine that contain more than one dose to prevent contamination and growth of potentially harmful bacteria.
- For children with a prior history of allergic reactions to any of these substances in vaccines, parents should consult their child's health-care provider.

What the Data Says About Vaccines

It is well documented that many of these additives cause severe reactions in children. According to the Vaccine Adverse Event Reporting System (VAERS) established by the FDA, vaccines are safe and complications only occur at an annual rate of one in one hundred thousand to one in one million.

I downloaded a spreadsheet directly from the VEARS website that listed an annual total of 45,742 reported vaccine reactions for 2016.[7] Ten to 15 percent of those reactions are classified as serious "(resulting in permanent disability, hospitalization, life-threatening illnesses or death)," according to the CDC. Some experts have estimated that only 40 percent of vaccine reactions are actually reported to the VEARS hotline so those numbers could actually be much higher.

The federal government does not allow lawsuits directly against pharmaceutical companies who manufacture vaccines. Lawsuits are directed to the federal government directly, which resulted in the creation of a trust fund called the *National Vaccine Injury Compensation Program* in 1988, specifically intended to compensate those who have suffered complications from vaccines. As of June 2016, over $2.8 billion has been awarded for vaccine injuries and deaths suffered by more than 4,500 children and adults, according to the US Government Accountability Office.

Looking Deeper

The chemicals that are added to vaccines are known to be toxic, especially to the brain and nervous system. Some data I reviewed claimed that mercury has been phased out as a preservative in most vaccines. Other data claims it is still used. Thimerosal is the mercury-based preservative that supposedly was removed from all vaccines except flu shots beginning in 1999. Yet there is still evidence in the literature that reviews the effects of thimerosal in current vaccines, such as DPT and MMR. Thimerosal is 50 percent ethyl mercury. Hair analysis of autistic children show a significant difference in mercury levels, .47 ppm (parts per million) versus 3.63 for ppm for non-autistic children, indicating autistic children are not excreting the mercury as efficiently as non-autistic children.[8] Granted, some of the mercury can come from other environmental sources including dental amalgam from the mother's teeth and from the mother's diet. Why is the mercury being excreted in some children more effectively than others?

In an adult, these chemicals are detoxified (removed) by glutathione. In a child, glutathione detoxification is inefficient through the first six years of life. In addition, some children have genetic SNiPs that prevent the methylation process from occurring, that regulates detoxification. Couple that with exposure to other drugs like acetaminophen, which is commonly given when a child develops a fever from a vaccine. It is well known that acetaminophen depletes glutathione from the body. This is comparable to throwing gasoline on a fire and then taking away the fire hose. Researchers have found a strong correlation between the onset of autism and aluminum exposure when it is coupled with the use of acetaminophen to combat fever.[9] Genetic SNiPs that impair methylation would dramatically increase the risk of complications since glutathione production is dependent on proper methylation.

The issue here is the repeated exposure of a child's immune system to chemicals that the child is not capable of handling. I have already discussed the harmful effects of MSG on the nervous system. If MSG is neurotoxic to an adult, rest assured it is neurotoxic to a child.

Aluminum is known to be toxic to specific areas of the brain and is strongly linked with Alzheimer's disease and other diseases. There is no safe level of aluminum consumption. Aluminum exposure induces significant production of free radicals that are well known to cause tissue destruction. Aluminum is now the chosen preservative to replace thimerosal. Take away the gasoline and add kerosene instead!

Clearly, when vaccines are given, there is more exposure for the child than just the vaccine. The truth is repeated exposure to these chemicals carries a significant risk of affecting a child's development. It is estimated that 673,000 US children have been diagnosed with autism. From 1960 to 1980, autism cases rose from one in five thousand to one in two thousand children (a 150 percent increase in twenty years). Studies in the early 2000s showed autism rates had increased dramatically to nearly one in 333 children. I have treated autistic children so I know firsthand the devastating effects this illness can bring to families.

When your child is one of the 40 percent who suffers a vaccine complication, it quickly becomes a significant issue that often ends up being a lifelong financial and emotional battle. It is estimated the lifetime health-care cost for a person with autism is more than $1.6 million. The total burden on the US health-care system for autism increased by 142 percent from the year 2000 to 2004 alone.[10, 11]

In addition to these factors, there is a wealth of evidence suggesting that prolonged vaccination regimens early in life combined with early use of antibiotics cause a shift in the immune system that causes diseases later in life. A normal-functioning immune system has a predominance of immunoglobulin G (IgG) in the bloodstream. IgG antibodies are the good guys as long as they are in proper balance. The immune system shift, referred to in the literature as the TH-1 >TH-2 shift, occurs when IgG transitions to IgE. IgE becomes the bad guy when it is overproduced. The predominant effect of over production of IgE is outlined below:

- High histamine release (allergies later in life)
- Asthma
- Eczema/psoriasis
- Autoimmune diseases (rheumatoid arthritis, lupus, Sjogren's disease, type 2 diabetes, multiple sclerosis)[12, 13]

Considering the evidence cited in chapter two for vitamin D improving the immune response, as well as the other citations for the damaging effects of sugar on the immune response, it would be well worth the effort to monitor these factors in children. In addition, the balancing effect of spinal adjustments and probiotics on the immune system is undeniable and could be considered as an alternative to routine immunization/antibiotic use. In my opinion, this could spare many families from the devastating effects of vaccines and antibiotics. Maybe someday research dollars will be provided to investigate this further.

Cancer-Causing Chemicals in the Environment

Chemical exposure is also in the surrounding environment. PBDEs (polybrominated diphenyl ethers) are used in everyday products like flame retardants that leach into the air and water. PBDEs are used in carpets, paint, bedding, mattresses, and some clothing. PBDEs are now considered ubiquitous; they can be found in the air, water, fish, birds, marine mammals, and even people. Unfortunately the oceans are becoming more contaminated with PBDEs which means people are being exposed to them in much higher amounts.

Every Day Foods Containing PBDE's and Other Contaminants

We commonly hear that eating fish is a healthy alternative to red meat. This notion is reinforced when you look at the data regarding fish consumption in the United States and from recommendations from the government:

Between 1987 and 1999, salmon consumption increased annually at a rate of 14 percent in the European Union and 23 percent in the United States. Over half the salmon sold globally is farm raised and labeled as Atlantic salmon.[14] *Farmed* salmon has a much higher concentration of PBDEs and other contaminants than wild caught salmon. Why? Because farmed salmon are routinely subjected to similar conditions as those of commercial chickens, i.e., overcrowding and disease infested fish pools treated with chemicals and antibiotics.[15] These contaminants tend to collect in the fat of the fish. This is unfortunate because farmed salmon has the potential to be a healthy source of nutrients if raised in a natural, uncontaminated environment.

Until recently the federal government has routinely recommended that people consume more fish, especially salmon, because it is high in omega-3 fatty acids. The previous guidelines failed to mention that most commercial sources of salmon are raised in fish farms. It has been documented that farmed salmon commonly contain high levels of PCBs, *methyl* mercury, dioxins and chlorinated pesticides. [16] Methyl mercury is the more potent cousin of ethyl mercury. This data caused the government to revise the guidelines on fish consumption.

The highest level of PCB exposure from fish occurred in farmed salmon sold from European fish farms. All Atlantic salmon comes from farmed sources. Salmon from all Atlantic waterways are protected species.[17] This means, salmon sold in stores and restaurants labeled as "wild Atlantic salmon" is either harvested illegally or they are being dishonest with their labeling. The reason for the higher concentrations of contaminants is believed to result from what the fish are being fed and severe overcrowding in fish hatcheries. Fish hatcheries are large barricaded pools of fish, located in the ocean waters.[18]

Toxic Fish

Studies have also concluded:

- "More than one 8-ounce portion of farmed salmon per month poses an unacceptable cancer risk to consumers."
- "It takes approximately three months for *one exposure* of methyl mercury to be removed from the body. It takes approximately eight years for PCBs to be removed from the body."
- "These contaminants are known to linger longer in the brain and kidneys than they are in the blood."
- Once the contaminants collect in the organs they become potent producers of free radicals.
- PBDE's are potent inhibitors of thyroid hormones, especially T4.

"Levels of mercury in fish continue to increase at approximately 4.8% per year." (That amount may go up significantly with the events that have been occurring worldwide. Since the 2013 nuclear reactor meltdown in Japan, the Pacific waterways, once known for being pure and pristine, now show high levels of "reactive contaminates," such as methyl mercury).

Other Facts Regarding Fish Consumption

Fish farms are creating problems for wild species of fish because the feed that is used in fish farms is known to contain toxic substances that leach out of the fish hatcheries into the ocean water. Wild species of fish are being contaminated from eating the toxic byproducts, including mercury. Even though it's not supposed to happen, crossbreeding of salmon from hatcheries and wild ocean salmon is also being observed, which is creating problems with genetic mutations in the fish.[19]

A healthy adult with efficient methylation pathways can excrete approximately 38.5 *micro*grams of mercury every two weeks. A 6oz. serving of swordfish can contain as much as 200 micrograms of mercury, more than five times the amount a healthy adult can excrete.[20] Friends, swordfish are *not* a farmed species of fish! These large fish species are absorbing mercury from the water in which they swim – the ocean. Yikes!

The most common farmed fish in the United States are:

1. Salmon
2. Tilapia
3. Catfish
4. Trout

The US Department of Agriculture reports that farmed salmon is by far the highest source of Arachidonic acid and other pro inflammatory chemicals in western diets, raising important questions regarding the safety of its consumption.[21] This is part of the new federal guidelines on fish consumption. Have you heard this anywhere? Even the government is now saying if you want to stay healthy you might want to avoid this stuff! Remember, AA is the chemical that produces PGE2, the number one cancer causing dietary chemical. How would fish contain AA when it's almost exclusively an animal based fat? It's because of the toxic soup the fish are being fed. Of all the species of salmon, Chinook was the highest in contaminants.

Regarding AA in other sources of fish; for a 3.5 oz. serving size:

- Central American farmed tilapia = 300mg of AA
- Farmed catfish = 67 mg of AA

In comparison to other foods:

- Pork bacon = 191 mg of AA
- Lean hamburger = 34 mg of AA

In other words, you're getting a larger dose of AA from salmon, tilapia and catfish than from eating a hamburger. Can you see why I said in chapter one that the diseases we are facing are self-inflicted? Not intentionally, but it is true and very unfortunate none-the-less.

What about tuna? Commercial tuna is yet another large ocean fish that is testing higher for mercury and PCB content. Tuna consumption is second in the US behind salmon. Years ago, many of my friends at the gym would eat several cans of tuna every day for its protein content. Regardless of its protein, tuna ranks at the very bottom of the list for its healthy omega 3 content (the good stuff). One can of commercial tuna yields approximately 65 micrograms of mercury. Remember the body can only excrete 38 micrograms every two weeks. This is very bad for sustaining health!

Oregon Fish Advisories

Toxic contaminants have become so bad in the state of Oregon that the Oregon Department of Human Services has issued warnings on consuming fish from sixteen of its lakes and streams. The contaminants listed in the warnings were: mercury, dioxins, PCB's and pesticides. Sound familiar? One can no longer assume fish caught from inland lakes and streams are automatically free from contaminants.[22]

Clinical Insight

You may ask how all this information relates to your routine care for common conditions. Can I give you a little clinical insight? Asthma is a common childhood and adult disease, accounting for approximately 12 percent of doctor visits annually. PGE2 is a potent chemical that can cause the airway constriction seen in asthmatics. However, asthmatics are also known to have high levels of the inflammatory chemical leukotriene B4 (LtB4) in their blood. The toxins contained in salmon and other fish are strong producers of PGE2 and LtB4, which means if you eat the salmon or other toxic fish it will make your asthma worse and can even trigger an asthmatic episode. In my experience, the etiology of asthma is usually assumed to be from inhaling environmental irritants. This information would suggest that dietary toxins play a major role in the etiology of asthma.

The medical treatment for asthma is corticosteroids or the epipen (epinephrine) in severe cases. These drugs relax the airways and help to ease the symptoms but they do nothing for lowering the PGE2 or LtB4 in the blood. If you suffer from asthma, you should be very careful about eating inflammatory foods: farmed fish, obese meat and refined carbohydrates. Reducing these foods and adding antioxidants and good omega 3 fats to your diet should help your asthma significantly.

Considering the many health-enhancing benefits of omega-3 fatty acids, eliminating them from the diet is a major mistake. An alternative is to take purified omega-3 oils in supplement form rather than relying exclusively on fish. If you do consume any fish, always verify that it is wild caught and not farm raised.[23] For now, it is safe to eat wild caught salmon, only if it's truly wild caught. Even then it would be safe to assume that limiting your fish consumption to one serving every two weeks might be advisable. If your methylation pathways are not operating efficiently it might be best to avoid fish altogether. A time may come in the not too distant future when even wild caught fish are unsafe for human consumption.

If you have reactions to fish you have probably discovered by trial and error what fish you can and cannot eat. Genetic SNiP testing can provide insight as to why you are sensitive to foods. Any physician can order the testing as long as state licensing allows it and the physician embraces the need for it. There are functional medicine doctors who can perform this testing for you.

High-Fructose Corn Syrup

I include a separate discussion on high-fructose corn syrup (HFCS) because it is an additive that has received media attention in recent years. You've seen the ads: "It's just like sugar." Two things make high-fructose corn syrup a dangerous food additive: One, it blocks insulin receptors, which regular sugar does not. This creates insulin resistance much faster than normal sugar. Two, it has been well documented that some forms of HFCS are manufactured using methyl mercury. The data is unclear regarding when, where, and how much mercury is used. Since mercury is strongly linked with brain development issues and one in five children are considered autistic, it would be wise to steer clear of any source of HFCS.[24]

The Heavy Hitters

Mass production of crops took a sharp increase in the early 1970s, thanks to government subsidies. Genetically modified seeds (GMOs) were also introduced for corn, wheat, and soy in 1970. A genetically modified seed is produced when the seeds of two or more crops are crossbred in a laboratory. The byproduct is no longer the same as the original seeds. By 2014, in the United States, 94 percent of the planted soybeans, 96 percent of cotton, and 93 percent of corn were genetically modified varieties. Corn, wheat, and soy are strong producers of Arachidonic acid. It took many years of research to determine that GMO corn, wheat, and soy contain higher concentrations of sugar than their non-GMO counterparts. Therefore, GMO corn, wheat, and soy produce higher amounts of AA in the body. If you remember, AA produces PGE2, the leading dietary cause of cancer, along with casein from milk. In other words, the wheat produced today is radically different from the wheat produced before 1970. This is the primary reason GMO seeds are being linked with higher rates of cancer. Before 1970, the incidence of wheat allergies and gluten intolerance was much less than today as well.[25, 26, 27]

This change in agricultural methods was a governmental recommendation to help feed a growing population and to help farmers stay viable. The change in methods led the American farmer to produce mostly corn, soy, and wheat rather than a wide variety of crops. Much of the explosion in inflammatory diseases can be traced back to this decision to subsidize these crops. Of course we didn't know then what we know now about the inflammatory effects of corn, wheat, and soy. We are still feeling the aftershocks from the US Department of Agriculture's fateful decision.

Another result of using GMO seeds was the need to use synthetic chemicals to protect the new form of crops. The synthetic chemicals that are sprayed on GMO crops have depleted vital nutrients from the topsoil of nearly every farm in America. In 1950, when organic farming was predominant, the average American farm had three feet of topsoil. Now the average farm has less than one foot of topsoil, which is where plants absorb their nutrients. Organic farming methods preserve the top-soil conditions to 1950s standards without the use of synthetic chemicals. Standard Process, a supplement manufacturer located in Palmyra, Wisconsin, uses organic farming exclusively to grow the crops used for its products. The company attests to the fact that all of its fields still have in excess of three feet of topsoil.

One of the many synthetic pesticides used in conjunction with genetically modified seeds is glyphosate. Glyphosate is absorbed when sprayed on the plant; thus, it can't be washed off before it is consumed. Genetically modified corn has been found to contain an average of 13 ppm (parts per million) of glyphosate; more than eighteen times the safe level of exposure set by the FDA.[28] Glyphosate use is still unrestricted in the United States but has been banned in many European countries.

There is a strong correlation between the introduction of GMO seeds, synthetic pesticides, and the explosion of degenerative disease in our society. According to researcher Dr. Stephanie Seneff, "Glyphosate is possibly the most important factor in the development of multiple chronic diseases and conditions that have become prevalent in Westernized societies." She continues, "Glyphosate is now associated with a long list of chronic illnesses, including autism, allergies, cardiovascular disease, cancer, obesity, depression, infertility, Alzheimer's disease, Parkinson's disease, and ALS, just to name a few."[29]

I agree with these statements; however, I would clarify that all toxins cause free radicals that lead to inflammation and chronic disease. Glyphosate is such a strong factor in the equation of chronic health because it is used in the production of so many foods consumed by the general population today.

Glyphosate has become yet another ubiquitous chemical in modern society. It is everywhere and in everything. The simple fact is, the body has a very difficult time detoxifying glyphosate because it destroys the detox pathways in the liver that break it down into nontoxic byproducts. These pathways detoxify many other chemicals as well, which are vital to maintaining health. Second, glyphosate destroys the natural flora (bacteria) in the gut that keeps our intestinal environment healthy. This has serious consequences for the body because the gut communicates with the brain! Disrupting this vital communication causes autism and the other diseases mentioned previously by Dr. Seneff. The volume of toxins we are exposed to can cause serious issues for the body. When toxins such as glyphosate inhibit the body from excreting them it becomes an even larger issue.

Toxic chemicals are part of everyday life. It's just a fact of the world in which we live. I have only presented a small fraction of the data on these potent toxins. Even though we can't escape from all chemicals, everyone should take steps to minimize their exposure. I say with all sincerity, anyone who ignores these recommendations does so at their own peril. It's that important! To start, buy organic whenever possible. This includes organic foods, bedding, and other household goods. I know there is a cost associated with organics but your health is worth it. Second, it is imperative that *everyone* consumes adequate supplementation to aid in detoxification and cell repair. Many of the nutrients that assist the body cell repair are difficult to obtain through diet alone.

CHAPTER 9

Methylation: The Key to Detoxifying the Body

By now, hopefully you have a better understanding of toxins and their profound effect on the body. Hopefully you also have noticed a reoccurring theme with many of these modern toxins: (1) they disrupt the endocrine system, and (2) they produce inflammation.

If your hormones cannot work effectively because the mitochondria and receptors are damaged, it is difficult to have a healthy body. This is simple anatomy and physiology. Yet I have read information from "authorities" who insist that the overall effect of these chemicals is negligible. One commentary talked about how researchers tested blood samples of large numbers of people and didn't find any traces of these toxins. This is the proverbial syndrome of "I can't see the forest because of the trees in front of me." The toxins that are not filtered and removed by the liver and kidneys are quickly stored in the body's organs and fat cells—after they have done their damage to the receptors and other vital cell components. If a large amount of toxins are in free circulation within the blood, we have a bigger problem because that would indicate the liver and kidneys are no longer filtering as they should. At that point there would be much more showing up in the blood than just the toxins.

The next important topic to understand is how to *detoxify* your body. There are methods of detoxification, such as colonics, colon flushes, infrared saunas, and fasting, that are valid ways to detoxify the body. I have used some of these with my family. These methods are beyond the scope of this book. If you detoxify using one of these methods, I strongly recommend seeking the guidance of a professional who is experienced in the method you are using.

The good news is the body has natural mechanisms that perform most of the detoxification automatically. One of those natural mechanisms is a process called methylation. The list of vital methylation functions is quite extensive. Here's a short list of those vital processes:

1. Removal of toxic substances from the body, i.e., heavy metals like lead, mercury, and other toxic chemicals.
2. Removal of hormones and neurotransmitters from the bloodstream after they have been utilized.
3. Proper energy production (ATP) in the mitochondria.
4. Maintaining healthy blood sugar.
5. Maintaining low levels of the inflammatory chemical homocysteine.
6. Proper DNA (gene) expression.
7. Production of the universal detoxifier glutathione.

Without proper methylation, none of these vital processes can take place in the body. The best way to maximize methylation is through regular consumption of green, leafy vegetables and cruciferous vegetables, such as broccoli and brussels sprouts. However, it is difficult to obtain sufficient amounts of nutrients from these foods to properly support methylation. The following antioxidants can be added to the diet to assist with proper methylation:

1. SAMe, along with B vitamins: B12, B 6, biotin, folic acid, niacin, and choline
2. N-acetyl cysteine
3. Curcumin

The most bioactive form of vitamin B12 and folic acid is the *methylated* form. The label will read "methylcobalamine" for vitamin B12. If the label says "cyanocobalamine," this version is not bioactive and therefore less effective. For the methylated version of folic acid, the label will read "5-methyl-tetrahydrofolate." The non-bioactive version of folic acid reads simply "folic acid" or "folate" on the label. Learning to read labels is very important when choosing the right supplements.

Genetic SNiPs

Genes are yet another example of the body's grand design. Of course we know that genes are passed down from our mother and father, but what are they and what do they do? Everyone has a slightly different genetic makeup. The purpose of our genes is to transmit information to other parts of the body in order to regulate that part of the body, whether it is regulating cell repair, detoxifying hormones, or producing energy (ATP). If we look inside our genes, they are actually strands of proteins called nucleotides. Different strands perform different functions. If we change one nucleotide in the strand, it completely changes the function of the gene. A gene SNiP (selective nucleotide polymorphism) occurs when a nucleotide is missing or changed which alters the function (expression) of the gene and thus alters the regulation of the body.

The MTHFR SNiP is one of many examples. It is estimated that 60-85 percent of the population has the MTHFR SNiP, which makes the body unable to methylate properly and thus unable to perform many of the vital functions stated on the previous page. Many people with type 1 and type 2 diabetes have the MTHFR methylation defect.[1] In this case, the diabetic condition can often be improved significantly with regular consumption of cruciferous vegetables and methylation-enhancing vitamins. I wonder how many diabetics have had the SNiP testing done.

Other facts about methylation include:

- Methylation is critically important to the genetic development of the brain.
- Approximately one third of DNA mutations that cause disease are attributed to problems with methylation.
- Methylation is a critical factor for gene expression and stopping genetic mutations.
- Methylation is the key factor for regulating a destructive protein called homocysteine. Elevated homocysteine levels are a marker for premature aging, premature death, free-radical damage, and more than one hundred diagnosed diseases.
- Some studies have linked elevated homocysteine with autism.[2]

I believe one of the major factors contributing to the rise chronic disease is due the damage to vital components of the cells, especially to the methylation pathways, from repeated exposure to toxins.

Vitamins: Necessary for Health or Waste of Money?

The vitamin industry has grown exponentially over the last ten to fifteen years in spite of a steady stream of negative publicity. It is now estimated that as much as 68 percent of Americans take vitamins on a regular basis.[3] People are reaching into their pockets and paying for nutritional supplements more than ever before. At the same time, new companies are appearing in the marketplace by the dozens, trying to capture their share of the wellness revolution. Even pharmaceutical companies have joined the vitamin craze. Are they really necessary? Are they safe? Let's take a look at this topic in more detail.

I have spent a good portion of my career studying, researching, and learning about new advances in nutritional supplementation. I have always recommended nutritional supplements to my patients. I am more convinced than ever before that supplements are a necessary part of staying healthy. There are many factors that have influenced my decision to recommend supplements to my patients, as well as take supplements myself.

As mentioned in chapter eight, soil conditions have become more depleted of nutrients as the use of genetically modified seeds and synthetic chemicals has been commercialized. In comparative analysis of the nutritional content of today's crops versus crops of the 1950s, studies have consistently shown a 25 to 40 percent loss in calcium, iron, phosphorus, protein, riboflavin, vitamin A, vitamin C, and other key minerals.[4] To put that into perspective, today it would take eight oranges to get the same vitamin A content of one orange in the 1950s. I wholeheartedly agree that we should try to get as much of our nutrition from whole foods as possible. However, the only way to do this is by eating organically grown foods or by growing your own organic food.

Natural Versus Synthetic

What is a synthetic vitamin? In essence it's a chemical that is formulated in a laboratory that mimics a real vitamin. Synthetic nutrients are similar in composition to a vitamin that is naturally contained in a whole food but differs from the whole food because it lacks the other cofactors that make up the whole food. It's these cofactors that give whole-food vitamins their power. The following effectively illustrates this point:

Approximately two to three times a year, a study will be published that challenges the notion that vitamins are beneficial for health. A 2013 study published in the *Journal of the National Cancer Institute* concluded that regular consumption of vitamin E was associated with an increased risk in cancer of the prostate in African-American men. However, in the study they reported using synthetic vitamin E instead of natural vitamin E. In my opinion, the outcome of this study was negatively influenced because of the decision to use synthetic versus natural vitamin E. Otherwise, I believe the study would have shown a decrease in prostate cancer. Why? Because this study conflicts with the results of other studies on vitamin E.[5]

Remember, antioxidants attenuate free radicals as inflammatory agents. So decreasing free radicals in any form should always decrease the risk of cancer. The researchers readily admitted in their conclusions that synthetic vitamin E was not the bioactive form of vitamin E. (*Bioactive* means the ability of the vitamin to do its job. The bioactive version is always the natural version.) They also specifically stated they were surprised at their findings, indicating they too expected to show a decrease in cancer relative to vitamin E intake. They commented that the dosage may have been a factor in the final outcome; i.e., the dosage may have been too high or too low. The final conclusion was that vitamin E consumption might actually increase the risk of prostate cancer. There was no comment on the possibility that a different outcome may have come from using natural vitamin E.

I remain suspicious that many researchers do not fully understand the difference in effectiveness between natural and synthetic vitamins. The good part of this study is it proves that synthetics are not true vitamins and are ineffective. Now they need to repeat the study using the natural form of vitamin E and even combinations of antioxidants.[6]

The other interesting thing in this study is that the researchers measured blood levels of omega-3 fats in all the participants, even though it was not a study on omega-3 fats. It's almost as if this was an afterthought to throw in at the last minute. They concluded that participants with the highest levels of omega-3 fats in their blood also had higher rates of cancer. Again this is a contradiction to what other studies have shown. However, the conclusion makes perfect sense considering synthetic vitamin E does not serve as a protective antioxidant. It is likely that these individuals were not consuming other antioxidants in their diet although the researchers did not specify that this was a measured part of the study. As I've said before, the research consistently states that consuming omega-3 oils without consuming an abundance of antioxidants increases your risk of cancer through oxidation of the oil.

> **Health Tip:** The body knows the difference between a natural and synthetic vitamin.

The diagram in figure 7 below represents the chemical composition of the entire vitamin C complex, and it supports my point on natural vs. synthetic vitamins. Most commercial vitamins use ascorbic acid as the source of vitamin C. In figure 7 you'll notice ascorbic acid is just one component of the vitamin C complex. The outer ring of the vitamin C complex is ascorbic acid, which is the antioxidant component. True vitamin C also contains flavonoids and other cofactors that contribute to its effectiveness as an antioxidant. The inner ring contains the vital cofactors that give vitamin C its power. Acerola berry and other fruits are examples of natural foods that contain the entire vitamin C complex. It is the natural foods containing the entire complex that are used for some natural vitamins.

Figure 7

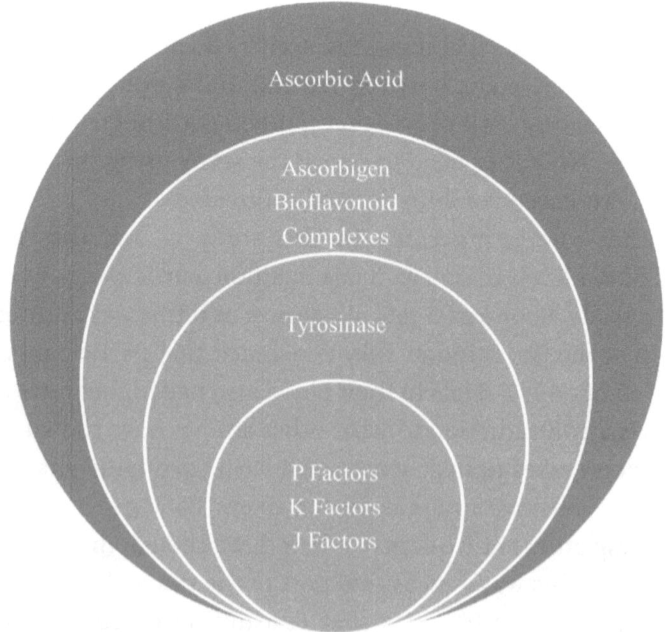

Vitamin C is composed of an outer layer of ascorbic acid (ascorbigen), along with a complex of nutrients called bioflavonoids. Ascorbic acid is the antioxidant component of vitamin C that is used in most commercial vitamin C. However, the diagram clearly shows ascorbic acid is only one component of the vitamin C complex. The remaining ingredients, shown above, also serve a vital role and are only found in natural or whole food versions of vitamin C.

It is unfortunate that most commercial vitamins are just a combination of synthetic compounds made in a laboratory. This is one reason why synthetics cost less than food-based vitamins. The person taking these vitamins does so without knowing that the ingredients in their vitamins are ineffective in nourishing and protecting the body, and in some cases they can actually cause more harm than good. At some point researchers use these products in their studies and conclude that vitamins cause disease. Synthetic compounds rarely produce positive actions in the body. The challenge for manufacturers is to maintain as much of the whole food value as possible when producing their supplements, even when individual nutrients are being extracted. This is not an easy thing to do and can result in additional cost. Likewise, the challenge for researchers is to be open to using natural sources of vitamins in their studies.

Health Tip: As a rule, if the source cannot be eaten in its natural form, don't expect the body to digest it.

Where Do Vitamins Come From?

Synthetic sources of vitamin C (ascorbic acid) and B vitamins are often extracted from coal tar. Calcium carbonate is extracted from oyster shells. Can coal tar and oyster shells be eaten raw? Of course not! These items can't be eaten in their natural form, so don't expect your body to get nutritional benefit from them. The nutrients are nonorganic and therefore essentially dead. Natural vitamins are made from pure food sources. Natural, food-based nutrients are made of living, organic complexes.

For example, carrots are high in vitamin A, so vitamin A can be extracted from carrots as a whole complex. It turns out that beta carotene is the antioxidant component of vitamin A, just as ascorbic acid is the antioxidant component of vitamin C. This is why most vitamin A is sold commercially as beta carotene. Actually there are hundreds of compounds called "carotenoids" that make up the whole vitamin A complex that you're not getting in the synthetic form. So when vitamin companies manufacture their products, they have a choice as to what sources will be used.

Another example of a food based vitamin is Citrus fruit. Citrus fruits are high in vitamin C, so vitamin C can be extracted from citrus fruits as a whole complex. This provides the entire vitamin C complex and not just synthetic ascorbic acid (see figure 7). And, wheat germ is high in vitamin E, so the vitamin E complex can be extracted from wheat germ. Vitamin E is a complex of compounds called tocopherols and tocotrienols. Synthetic vitamin E is made of strictly the laboratory-derived version of alpha tocopherol called dl-alpha tocopherol. This is the version that was used in the prostate cancer study cited earlier.

Most commercial vitamins on the shelves of your local supermarket are made from synthetic ingredients, and the tablets are bound together so tightly using binders and fillers that it becomes more difficult for the body to break down the tablet in the digestive tract. In my experience, the results are much better with natural vitamins. I have seen this time and time again in clinical practice. When better sources are used, the results improve too. Although this has been my clinical experience in recommending vitamins to patients, it is difficult to prove nonetheless because there are limited studies to support this conclusion.

Dosage

Most of what we read in terms of dosage for vitamins is considered textbook dosages based upon averages. I often tell patients, "Your body didn't study the textbook" when it comes to dosage. Sometimes it takes larger quantities of nutrients for a short time period to bring your body into balance. Likewise, some people only require a small fraction of the traditional "recommended daily allowance" (RDA) of certain nutrients.

The following is a partial list of helpful vitamins and nutrients:

1. Antioxidants. Think of the acronym ACES.
   A—vitamin A (minimum 3000 IU)
   C—vitamin C (minimum 150 mg)
   E—vitamin E (minimum 400 IU)
   S—selenium (minimum 50 µg)

2. CoQ10 (minimum 100 mg)
3. Alpha lipoic acid (minimum 50 mg)
4. Acetyl L-carnitine (minimum 100 mg)
5. Vitamin D in adequate amounts to maintain blood levels (between 50 and 70 mg/dL).
6. A quality omega-3 oil supplement, such as fish oil, containing EPA\DHA (2.5 g minimum); a supplement like flax seed oil (100 mg) containing ALA; and a GLA source, such as blackcurrant seed oil or borage oil (100 mg).

   Warning: Make sure the oil is purified of contaminants as it is processed. Consuming an unpurified source of fish oil is not recommended due to the high level of contaminants (PCBs, methyl mercury) inherent in most sources of fish oil. Always couple your dose of fish oil with plenty of antioxidants, especially vitamin E. Fish oil is easily oxidized, even from exposure to sunlight. Free radicals within the body will oxidize omega-3 oils. Oxidized fish oil becomes rancid and acts as a carcinogen (cancer-causing agent) once it is consumed.
7. Probiotics. There is a wealth of evidence connecting the health of the gut to a healthy immune system and a healthy brain. Be sure to include a wide spectrum of good bacteria, including L. acidophilus, L. bulgaricus, and bifidus factor. Different bacteria colonize in different areas of the intestines. People commonly tell me they are taking probiotics only to find out they are taking only acidophilus. This is not adequate to support intestinal health.
8. Glutathione is considered the universal detoxifier. It must be manufactured in the liver and requires specific nutrients in the diet that are commonly deficient. Toxic heavy metals are removed from the body with glutathione. Glutathione is very inefficient in children, which makes them especially vulnerable to injury from toxic exposure. It is difficult to raise glutathione levels because it is poorly absorbed when taken orally. The best way to raise glutathione levels is by taking N-acetyl cysteine in supplement form. Studies have shown that undenatured whey protein also raises glutathione levels. Most of the commercial whey protein on store shelves is "whey protein isolate," which is chemically treated to be "predigested." Unfortunately, this form of whey does not raise glutathione levels. It also has the potential to be an excitotoxin

> that damages nerve cells, according to Dr. Blaylock. People who take whey protein isolate would get more benefit by switching to undenatured whey. The benefits are much greater with less chance of toxic effects.[7] Whey protein concentrate is acceptable, but I believe the research suggests that the best support for glutathione production comes from undenatured whey.

This number of supplements may seem excessive until you consider the toxic world in which we live. I consider it a part of living in the twenty-first century with all of its pro-inflammatory toxins. Otherwise our bodies are sitting ducks to these toxins. Many of these nutrients cannot be derived from food alone.

In my clinical experience, I have observed that the body does not always absorb 100 percent of the nutrients in foods or supplements. Sometimes this is by design. Sometimes it's due to internal problems. For example, calcium is normally absorbed in a small portion of the upper small intestine (duodenum). Therefore, only one-third of the calcium that is ingested is absorbed in the bloodstream. Even then, if stomach acids are lacking from over consuming antacids, it can decrease calcium absorption even further. The same can be said for B vitamins, iron, and other nutrients, which are absorbed in specific regions of the digestive tract.

Absorption of these nutrients in this fashion is by design. Proper absorption is a delicate balance of factors that can ultimately be altered by unhealthy habits. Inflammatory conditions such as leaky gut syndrome, often caused by overconsumption of processed food, causes an overgrowth of foreign bacteria in the intestine. This will significantly reduce the absorption of nutrients. Therefore, it may require higher amounts of vitamins and minerals to achieve appropriate results. This is an internal physical problem that needs to be corrected in order to have proper absorption.

Additional Precautions about Copper and Iron in Vitamins

When taking vitamins, it's important to know what is in them. Copper and iron are commonly added to many commercial vitamins. They are necessary minerals in trace amounts, but in excess they are known to produce free radicals. Copper and iron from food sources such as red meat, almonds, cashews, pistachios, and other nuts contain an organically bound copper that quickly becomes stored in the liver. Thus, it is rendered harmless. Inorganic copper comes from most commercial supplements, municipal drinking water supplies, and copper pipes used in many older homes. This form of copper is not organically bound, thus it bypasses the liver and enters the bloodstream directly, increasing the chances for production of free radicals. Inorganic copper has been shown to collect in key areas of the brain, and copper toxicity has been strongly considered a contributing factor for Alzheimer's disease. [8] Because copper and iron are present in common foods like almonds and cashews, it is not necessary to consume these minerals in supplement form.

Regarding iron intake, there may be a few exceptions to the rule to limit intake of iron. One of those exceptions is for menstruating females who become anemic from the loss of blood during their cycles. Only in rare cases is it necessary to consume additional iron because the liver stores large quantities of it. When iron levels drop during the menstrual cycle, the liver will release more iron into the bloodstream. People who continually find themselves anemic should seek the advice of a health-care provider before taking iron supplements due to their high free-radical activity.[9]

There is even evidence that antioxidants and B vitamins help to preserve specific parts of the DNA strands called telomeres, believed to be a representation of a person's biological age. Shortened telomeres are strongly linked with accelerated aging and chronic disease. However, high iron intake is associated with shortened telomere length. [10] Watch your multivitamins for copper and iron content.

CHAPTER 10

pH: A Vital Link to Better Health

Most of us have heard of the term "pH" before, but some may be confused about what it means and why it is important to overall health. We have pH-balanced shampoos and hygiene products, pH-balancing fertilizers for crops, etc. Many other examples could be listed. Science defines *pH* as "potential of hydrogen" because acid is produced in all liquids from the accumulation of hydrogen ions. More hydrogen ions means more acid is produced; less hydrogen ions means less acid is produced. First, let's understand the basics of pH before we get into pH of the body.

The scale that measures pH spans from zero to fourteen. Zero is extremely acid; fourteen is extremely alkaline. Figure 8 is a visual representation of the pH scale. Battery acid in your car has a pH of about two. Ammonia is said to be alkaline because it has a pH of about eleven. Pure water has a neutral pH of seven.

Figure 8: The pH Scale

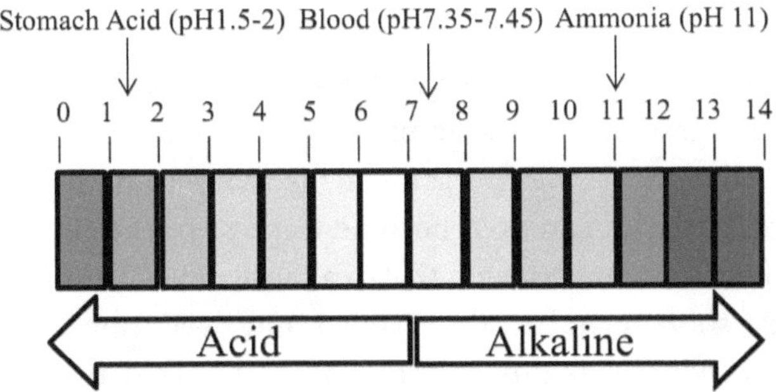

The numbers on the pH scale can be a little deceiving because the scale is logarithmic. As a result, each whole pH value below seven is ten times more acidic than the next higher value. For example, pH 4 is ten times more acidic than pH 5 and one hundred times (ten times ten) more acidic than pH 6. The same holds true for pH values above seven, each of which is ten times more alkaline than the next higher whole number. For example, pH 10 is ten times more alkaline than pH 9 and one hundred times more alkaline than pH 8.

pH and Body Fluids

The environment inside and outside the cells is mostly fluid and minerals (electrolytes). The pH of this fluid is said to mirror the pH of the blood. Notice in figure 8 that blood has a pH that is slightly alkaline at 7.35 to 7.45. What seems like a minimal variance is actually a tenfold change going from 7.35 to 7.45. Since the body is 75 percent water and water contributes to blood plasma, the pH of most body fluids tends to fall in this range as well. There are a few notable exceptions. The pH of the digestive tract varies widely depending on the location as described below:

- Saliva—considered the first stage of digestion. Contains a large amount of enzymes and is generally slightly alkaline.
- Stomach acid—proteins like meat or chicken require more acid (pH 2–3) than vegetables and fruits (pH 3–4).
- Bile—usually has a pH of 7–8 depending on the type of food digested.

Note: Digestion is most efficient at these pH ranges. If the stomach's pH is not acidic enough to break down proteins, indigestion and heartburn are the end result. Most heartburn issues are caused by an overall lack of acidity in the stomach, causing incomplete breakdown of the proteins as they pass through the digestive tract. This produces putrefaction (rotting) of the proteins, producing strong inorganic acids that can irritate the stomach lining. Small particles can even become trapped in the tiny spaces of the stomach, which ferments bacteria that can cause ulcers. This is why antacids only provide short-term heartburn relief and over time will worsen the problem. Antacids are alkaline salts that neutralize acid, including stomach acid necessary for digestion.

In my experience, chronic heartburn is often a result of improper nerve supply from the spine to the stomach, pancreas and liver, which can be fixed through chiropractic adjustments and digestive enzymes supplemented to assist the body in breaking down food. This is the reason so many people suffering from heartburn report significant improvements in their digestion when they take a tablespoon of apple cider vinegar with each meal. It enhances digestion. If apple cider vinegar causes heartburn to worsen, this is a strong indicator of a stomach ulcer. In this case I would suggest seeking the advice of a holistic doctor such as a chiropractor who practices with an emphasis in nutrition or a naturopath to help heal the ulcer.

Buffers in the Blood

Even though the digestive tract has some variation in pH, the body always makes adjustments to bring the pH of the blood and cellular fluid back to its normal range of 7.35 to 7.45. The pH of the blood affects the ability of the red blood cells to carry oxygen. In general, the oxygen capacity of red blood cells is greatest when the pH of the blood is at 7.4 to 7.45 and is reduced as the blood becomes more acidic. Various forms of free radicals are produced if red blood cells cannot carry enough oxygen to supply the body's needs, a condition called hypoxia.[1] Maintaining proper blood pH has a direct bearing on limiting free-radical production. It is important that the pH of the body stays in this narrow range; otherwise, the organs can quickly become damaged. Complete organ failure can result in severe cases if the pH becomes too high or too low. Chronic hypoxia has been linked with numerous chronic diseases, including heart disease, autoimmune disorders, and kidney disease.[2, 3]

Even though the body functions best in a slightly alkaline environment, the cells produce acid as a byproduct of metabolism. What a beautiful representation of grand design. The body always has counterbalancing mechanisms that keep things in their proper place. In this case the mechanism that balances acid in the blood is called a buffer. The primary buffer in the bloodstream is sodium bicarbonate. Sodium bicarbonate helps to maintain the blood's pH by absorbing or releasing acid. As you can see from the words *sodium* and *bicarbonate*, the body uses minerals in the diet, especially sodium, to buffer acid in the blood. We hear so much about salt restriction, but a certain amount of sodium, especially from fruits and vegetables, is actually beneficial to the body. There is not an infinite supply of minerals in the body so they must be replenished through the diet. We give a boost to the buffer systems by eating a diet that is centered on alkalizing foods. This is helpful to know because the standard American diet is heavily centered on acidifying foods that stress the body's buffer systems. This is why it is also helpful to know which foods are acidic and which foods are alkaline.

Balancing Acid and Alkaline Foods

I mentioned in the introduction that the body is like a garden because both must be nurtured to get the maximum benefit. Eating healthy is just one of the many ways in which we create the conditions inside the body that assure maximum health. The foods you eat on a daily basis are creating the conditions inside your body that either sustain health or enhance disease. We may not think of it in that context, but it's true. On one hand it is empowering to know that we are able to influence our health by what we eat and drink. On the other hand, it can be overwhelming to know this if we don't know the basic factors involved. Remember my reference to the roadmap at the beginning of the book? This is a major part of the roadmap. The reasons for not eating properly can be multifaceted, but the end result is still the same. Poor diet leads to poor health regardless if it's done because of limited finances (can't afford healthy food), no time for proper meal planning, or lack of knowledge regarding a balanced diet.

A balanced diet must contain a generous portion of alkalizing vegetables and fruits to offset the acid that is produced from proteins and stressful thinking. Therefore, a balanced diet will naturally help to maintain the pH of your body. An unbalanced diet and overconsumption of acid-producing sodas will cause stress to your liver and kidneys. It's that simple. Before I get into the basics of what a proper diet looks like, it would be helpful for you to understand some basics about pH and how it relates to diet.[4]

As a general rule, pH is strongly influenced by the "ash" that is left over *after* the digestion process is completed. Most vegetables and some fruits are considered "alkaline ash" foods, meaning they *alkalize* the body. Proteins are considered "acid ash" foods, meaning they *acidify* the body. Many people get confused on this topic of acid versus alkaline. The mineral content of vegetables and the alkaline ash that is left over from the digestion process is what alkalizes the body. Citrus and many other fruits are *acidic* before they are digested. However, citrus *alkalizes* the body because the ash that is left over after digestion is alkaline. Therefore, citrus is considered an alkaline ash fruit. Likewise it's the high content of hydrogen ions in proteins that acidifies the body. This is important information to keep in mind in balancing your food choices.

Proteins, especially dairy products and meat products, are acid producing. The standard American diet that is promoted as being healthy is heavily concentrated in the acid-producing category. Eating too much protein over long periods can damage the kidneys and liver. Currently the recommended daily allowance (RDA) for protein stands at 52 and 55 grams for females and males, respectively. An omelet, potatoes, and toast for breakfast will have about 30–35 grams of protein. Add chicken salad for lunch and pot roast for dinner, and you could easily be pushing 75–100 grams for the rest of the day. This is more than the body needs for daily consumption of protein unless you're a training athlete. But it gives you an idea of how quickly protein intake can exceed even the recommended daily allowance.

Lastly, stress is a strong producer of acid in the body. In fact the strongest acid generator within the body is stress. Stress management and proper diet are the key factors in maintaining a healthy pH. Junk food not only causes free-radical production but also acidifies the body, which places tremendous stress on the organs.

The Basics of a Balanced Diet

There is a wealth of information on the beneficial effects of an antioxidant-rich diet. I have included some interesting references at the end of this chapter on the health benefits of various fruits and vegetables. We have seen the importance of antioxidants in neutralizing free radicals in previous chapters. Antioxidants also maintain proper pH of the body.

Antioxidants come from vegetables and fruit with color. Green, leafy vegetables and cruciferous vegetables, such as broccoli and brussels sprouts, are packed with antioxidants and phytonutrients, plant-based nutrients that are only derived from vegetables and certain fruits. Many phytonutrients have powerful cancer-fighting properties. Some phytonutrients help with detoxification and aid in balancing hormones. Raspberries and blueberries have been widely studied for their antioxidant content, but blueberries in particular have been shown to have strong protective effects against cancer and vascular disease, and even promote brain health. An abundance of these foods is extremely beneficial to the body. The only caution on fruit consumption is for people who have blood sugar problems. In this case, try to limit your fruit consumption to no more than two cups per day. If your blood sugar is staying within a normal range at this level, it may be acceptable to increase that number slightly. If you make these changes, you will maximize your body's ability to detoxify unwanted substances, as well as maximize healing and cell repair.

Tables 5 and 6 list some common acid and alkaline ash foods. Keep in mind, just because a food item is listed as alkaline or acid does not mean that item should not be consumed. The key here is moderation. Olive oil, for example, is listed as acid producing, but olive oil is still healthy and has many health-enhancing benefits. Some of the heavy acid producers, such as grass-fed meat and certain white fish, are still health enhancing even though they are on the acid side of the scale. Just make sure to balance acid producers with alkaline producers. That is your goal every day in balancing your food choices.

Table 5.

Alkaline Ash Foods			
Apples	Cauliflower	Limes	Raisins
Apricots	Celery	Molasses	Raspberries
Avocado	Cucumbers	Mushrooms	Raw spinach
Bananas	Dried beans	Oranges	Rutabagas
Beets	Dried dates	Onions	Sour cherries
Blackberries	Dried figs	Parsnips	Strawberries
Blueberries	Grapes	Peaches	Sweet potatoes
Broccoli	Grapefruit	Pears	Tangerines
Brussels sprouts	Green beans	Peas	Tomatoes
Cabbage	Lemons	Pineapple	Watermelon
Carrots	Lettuce	Radishes	Watercress

Table 6.

Acid Ash Foods			
Bacon	Eggs	Pasta noodles	Sugar
Beef	Fresh corn	Peanuts	Turkey
Brown rice	Haddock	Pike fish	Veal chops
Chicken	Honey	Pork chops	Walnuts
Cod fish	Lamb	Salmon	Wheat bread
Corn beef	Lobster	Sausage	Wheat flour
Corn oil	Oatmeal	Scallops	Wheat germ
Corn syrup	Olive oil	Shrimp	White bread
Dried lentils	Oysters	Soda Crackers	White flour

On the surface it may seem overly simplistic to say that lifestyle changes can prevent cancer, heart disease, strokes, and Alzheimer's disease, but it's really not an oversimplification at all. Some research articles I have referenced in this book have commented that even moderate changes in dietary habits can bring profound improvements in overall health.[5] It just takes a concerted effort to change lifestyle habits that many times span back for generations. Sedentary lifestyles, over consuming processed foods, and toxic exposure are the enemies that are eroding our health. Begin by making small changes. The benefits will speak for themselves over time.

There are some very good diet plans out there, such as the Paleo diet and the Mediterranean diet. Following these plans will lead you back to the same diet recommendations I have made in this book. Here are some general guidelines to follow for improving your diet:

1. Limit sweets and junk food.
2. Reduce intake of refined oils and processed foods.
3. Increase intake of fresh, organic vegetables and fruit.
4. Red meat is fine in moderation as long as the meat is grass fed, organic, and hormone-free. Poultry is fine as well, as long as it is free range, chemical free, and vegetarian fed.
5. If you eat fresh fish, always try to find wild caught sources of fish. Wild caught fish are much less likely to be contaminated with PCBs and toxic metals.

Balance is the key for a proper diet. In general, always strive for a balance of 60 percent vegetables and fruits, 30 percent protein and good fats, and 10 percent nuts and seeds.

Cooked vegetables are fine as long as they are lightly steamed or sautéed so they have some crunch left in them. The crunchiness in the prepared vegetables indicates all of the nutrition has not been cooked out of them. Remember, vegetables and fruits are at the core of these diets because these foods have the highest concentrations of disease-fighting vitamins, minerals, and antioxidants. Combine them with smaller portions of quality proteins and essential fats, and you have a recipe for healthy living that maintains the body's natural processes, which includes having a balanced pH.

There is an old proverb that says "let food be your medicine." There are times when our culture has nearly reversed that proverb to say "let medicine be your food." In my practice, I have frequently encountered patients who were advised to refrain from taking fish oil, antioxidants, and other health-enhancing products because they conflict with their medications. Avoiding interaction between products is one thing but withholding vital nutrients that are health sustaining is quite another.

I believe we are seeing a gradual transition back to the foundation of healing through diet, herbs, plants, and vitamins. This is evidenced by the massive volume of scientific literature that supports the health-enhancing properties of foods, herbs, and vitamins. It is so extensive that I could fill an entire book with those references. There may have been a time in history when the benefits of these things had not been studied and were not well understood. That is not the case today. The more we understand about the healing power of specific foods, the more we can utilize those foods as potential healing agents in chronic disease and the preservation of wellness.

Two prime examples are blueberries and carrots. Both are considered powerhouses of nutrition for various reasons. The antioxidants in blueberries have been shown to inhibit heart disease, improve kidney function, reduce oxidative stress, reduce inflammation, stabilize blood pressure, prevent Alzheimer's disease, and even protect from certain types of cancer. There is even evidence that the anti-inflammatory properties of blueberries prevent inflammation in an unborn child. Raspberries have similar healing properties.[6,7] Although carrots have taken their fair share of criticism because of their high natural sugar content, carrot juice has been shown to have protective properties when the body has been exposed to inflammation induced by consumption of fructose from other sources, such as high-fructose corn syrup.[8] This implies carrot juice may have other protective properties for the body that may be worthy of future research studies.

The key point to understand here is that diets high in fruits, vegetables, and micronutrients can help prevent many types of disease and even show benefits when certain diseases already are present.[9, 10] This is the true definition of "let food be your medicine," which makes pharmaceuticals much less necessary.

Making Dietary Changes

If you find yourself thinking that you will start changing your diet next week, next month, next year, let me give you some thoughts to ponder. One study conducted on 12 healthy college age men has shown that changes occur in the blood very quickly with consistent intake of processed food. After one week of a diet consisting of macaroni and cheese, processed lunchmeat, sausage, biscuits, mayonnaise, and microwavable meals with unhealthy fats, their bodies were already showing signs of losing the ability to metabolize glucose, seen with insulin resistance.[11] Another study showed a strong correlation between dietary PGE2 (in this case from farmed fish) and significant irreversible aggregation (clumping) of platelets, a significant risk factor seen in stroke patients.[12]

Think about this for a minute: according the U.S. Department of Health and Human Services, there are currently 6 million people taking blood thinners at an annual cost of 1 billion dollars. The reason so many people are taking blood thinners is because their blood is too thick, which causes an unstable heart rhythm (arrhythmia). The blood collects in the arteries and forms clots. Indeed, these individuals are at high risk for a stroke without the medication. However, if you recall, in chapter 5 I discussed the benefits of omega 3 therapy. Among their many benefits, omega 3's stabilize heart rhythm, they thin the blood, and they are anti-inflammatory. The reason so many people are having issues with excessive blood clotting is because of the epidemic of inflammation throughout our culture, combined with significant deficiencies of magnesium and other vital nutrients. This is why it is so important to take charge of your health by insisting on having your inflammatory markers tested. In review, they are: AA/EPA ratio, c-reactive protein, homocysteine, insulin and VLDL (very low density lipoproteins). Unfortunately, routine testing of these markers is not a part of the current and accepted protocol, even though there is a wealth of information to support them in the literature.

Change is difficult if you don't know your destination or your map is pointing you in the wrong direction.

When contemplating making changes, the assumption is usually that I'll be healthy when I get around to it. If one week of refined food can cause early insulin resistance in otherwise healthy men, how many meals will it take to cause more severe problems? If your blood is already inflamed from PGE2 and free radicals, it could be the next meal that causes a heart attack or a stroke. These studies raise serious doubts about that assumption and add strong ammunition to not delay what you can and should do today.

CHAPTER 11

Conclusion

One of the greatest examples of Gods grand design is the human nervous system. We know the nervous system communicates with every cell in the body. This makes perfect sense because the primary job of the nervous system is to regulate the function of all other systems. It would make no sense at all for the master control center to have parts of the body that are not in direct communication with the systems that it controls. With that said, there is a spark of creative intelligence that flows through every nerve that tells the cell exactly what, where, when and how to perform its job. Without this spark, life ceases to exist. Chiropractors call this "innate intelligence." Innate intelligence is inborn within every human that has ever lived and ever will live, past, present and future. At its core, innate intelligence is truly a spark of divine spirit that creates all living cells. The Bible clearly says God is the creator of all things.

The beauty in God's grand design is in the fact that your body was created with systems in place that are designed to manage the toxic exposure. Without these systems your body would never have made it this far. Like all good things, the body has limitations. Chiropractor's call this "limitations of matter." If you recall, I quoted scripture in chapter one that expresses this point exactly: "God has appointed his limits that man cannot exceed." The next verse does not say this directly but I believe it could be: "if you exceed these limits there will be consequences."

I reviewed volumes of literature during the course of writing this book and I probably left out more than I included. It became clear to me very early that what we are seeing on a wide scale is the detoxification pathways of the body becoming overwhelmed. I have heard it said that the difference between order and chaos is a fine line. There is a tipping point in which the body ceases to reproduce healthy cells and begins to produce diseased cells. The tipping point is usually when the body loses the ability to adapt to its environment. For example, repeated exposure to toxins producing inflammation, causing the production of free radicals and over stimulating the immune system as described in chapter four. Still, the body can overcome this if the toxic exposure ceases. However, if toxic exposure continues, day after day, month after month, the cells of the body begin to break down. Everyone has a slightly different ability to heal. Some people can overcome the effects of significant, prolonged unhealthy choices. Some people are overwhelmed with health issues much sooner.

The emphasis in this book is to be proactive and not wait until you feel bad to think about prevention. The things you have read in this book regarding toxins, inflammation and free radicals are a clear representation of the body becoming overwhelmed and losing the ability to adapt to its environment, thereby causing disease. Here's another key: *The spine takes the brunt of these stresses.* The nerves connecting the brain to the body are an absolutely critical aspect of keeping the body healthy. Research has even suggested that one is only as healthy as their spine. I have seen this repeatedly in my years of clinical practice. Don't underestimate the power of the things that are within your control, including spinal hygiene through regular spinal adjustments and improving your diet.

I can say with absolute certainty that, even though we know a lot about disease prevention, there is still much to learn. Diet, nutrition and exercise are powerful things, no doubt about it. Indeed, they are the very foundation of health. However, I also know for certain that the best nutrition in the world will not turn off the stress response coming from our own mind. I touched on this in chapter four with a discussion on the mind-body connection. I have witnessed the powerful impact of stress and the toll it takes on the human frame (body structure) of patients every day in my practice. The negative impact on the body structure plays a major role in producing chronic inflammation which can have devastating consequences if left uncorrected. Chronic inflammation is difficult to control under high levels of stress that induce harmful changes to the nervous system and body frame, especially the spinal column.

As time goes by, it becomes clearer to me that unless we find better ways to manage stress, improving our diets and exercise will only be addressing part of the puzzle. And the part that is left, the stress response of the body has the power to negate even the best nutritional protocols.

There is a positive side that should not be overlooked. Research data and clinical observations support the conclusion that chiropractic adjustments have far-reaching, positive effects on balancing the nervous system and easing chronic inflammation. [1,2] After one hundred-plus years, this still seems to be a little known secret, known only to the ones who have experienced the benefits of chiropractic firsthand. Even with limited funding for research, the advances that have been made in chiropractic are on the cutting edge of mind-body medicine. I plan to share more information about this in future books. But for now, I hope this information stirs within you a quest for knowledge.

I conclude with a few of my favorite case studies from my years in practice. This is just a small sample of lives that were changed through the power of the chiropractic adjustment. Hopefully you too will experience these benefits in your quest for better health. God bless!

Case Studies

The following case histories are typical representations of the situations I would see in everyday practice. The cases are real although names have been changed for privacy. The common theme of these cases is that the cause of the patients' problems was related to structural imbalances (subluxations). I didn't have to name the disease in order to treat the root of the problem. Structure and function are directly related. Never forget that.

Case #1

Anna was eight months old when her mother, Christine, brought her into my office. Case history revealed that Anna had been severely constipated since birth. It was not unusual for her to go for seven to ten days without a bowel movement. Anna was colicky and seldom slept through the night. Christine informed me that her pediatrician had said seven to ten days between bowel movements was just normal for Anna. He recommended putting Metamucil in her formula, which only served to make her even more colicky.

Constipation is usually related to subluxations at the atlas (the first vertebra below the skull) or the pelvis. On examination, I found that Anna did indeed have a subluxation of the atlas, which was adjusted. I also balanced her energy through a specialized technique. I told Christine that Anna should have a bowel movement within the next six to eight hours. Christine and Anna left for the day, and I resumed seeing the rest of my patients.

About ninety minutes later, my chiropractic assistant knocked on my office door and informed me that Christine was on the phone and needed to speak to me "urgently." When I got to the phone, Christine told me in a half-excited, half-panicked tone that Anna had a large bowel movement even before they arrived home. Christine no sooner got Anna's diaper changed than she had another bowel movement. She changed Anna again and went about her business. About twenty minutes later, she returned to find that Anna once again had filled her diaper.

It was only after changing her third diaper that Christine decided to call me to find out if this was okay or if something was wrong. I assured Christine that it was perfectly normal and it would take a day or two for Anna's bowels to regulate completely. When Christine returned in two days, she informed me that Anna had slept through the night both nights after her first adjustment. She also had normal bowel movements twice on both days. I adjusted Anna two more times before placing her on maintenance care, where she would be checked once a month. Her problems with constipation were completely resolved, as well as her inability to sleep at night.

Case #2

John is a thirty-two-year-old male who entered my office with a complaint of lower back pain radiating into his right leg. His family doctor had previously sent him to a neurosurgeon. The neurosurgeon ordered an MRI on his lower back, which showed that John had a bulging disc at the L5 level. The neurosurgeon recommended surgery as soon as possible. A friend of John's, who was a patient of mine, suggested that John should see me before having surgery. It should be noted that the neurosurgeon told John *not* to consult a chiropractor because in his opinion a chiropractor could not help with his condition.

On examination, I found that John had subluxations in the neck, mid back, lower back, and pelvis. Adjustments were immediately administered to begin the process of fixing the subluxations in his spine. After the third adjustment, his leg pain had subsided although he still had some back pain, but it was less severe. After the sixth adjustment, his back pain was barely noticeable. After the tenth adjustment, his back pain was completely gone. John had also experienced daily headaches, which resolved completely as well.

I placed John on a comprehensive program of adjustments, stretches, and exercises to correct his subluxations. After the corrective care was completed, John was placed on monthly wellness adjustments. He never had back pain after that tenth visit. Incidentally, when John returned to his neurosurgeon and informed him that he did see a chiropractor and was 100 percent better, the neurosurgeon told him that his back pain would return and still recommended surgery. John refused the neurosurgeon's advice and chose to continue with chiropractic as a part of a holistic wellness plan.

Case #3

Tammy and her husband had been trying to conceive for approximately four years with no success. She had been through twelve months of fertility treatment, which only served to make her moody and depressed. So a friend of Tammy's, who also was a patient of mine, referred her to my office. Tammy told me she did not have high hopes that my treatment would be successful, but she was willing to give it a try.

On examination I found that Tammy had subluxations in the neck and pelvis. The subluxation in her pelvis was severe and was causing her uterus to tilt. I had a strong suspicion that this was the source of her fertility problems. We began an immediate care plan to correct her subluxations. After about two months of treatment, Tammy entered my office one day with a smile of joy on her face. She informed me that she was pregnant. She carried the baby full term and delivered a healthy baby girl eight months later.

Case #4

Tom is a thirty-two-year-old male who was referred to my office for evaluation of multiple complaints. Tom suffered from bipolar disorder for most of his adult life. During that time he had received traditional psychiatric care in the form of counseling and psychotropic medications. He reported occasionally feeling suicidal. At the time of consultation,

Tom's medication list included Neurontin, lithium, and Klonopin. He had recently taken Seroquel and Wellbutrin. In addition to bipolar disorder, Tom experienced frequent headaches, fatigue, irritability, insomnia, and general malaise that made it difficult for him to sustain long-term employment.

Further questioning of Tom's dietary and lifestyle habits revealed that his diet consisted of mostly fast food. He had periods in the past where he was active and exercised regularly, but these were not a part of his current routine.

An examination revealed subluxation patterns in his neck, mid back, and pelvis. Tom was placed on a care plan of adjustments and lifestyle modifications that included reduced consumption of fast food in favor of vegetables, fruit, and whole foods. Daily exercise was recommended as well as whole food supplements, broad-spectrum B vitamins, and SAMe for assistance in his methylation pathways. After one week of adjustments and lifestyle modifications, Tom reported significant improvements in his sleep patterns, his mood, and his energy levels. No headaches were reported after his second treatment. After only seven treatments, Tom showed significant improvement in all of his symptom patterns.

This was following one week of care with seven treatments. Tom will require additional care, but this emphasizes the significant impact dietary changes, exercise and chiropractic adjustments can make relatively quickly. It should be noted no changes were made to his prescribed medications.

In Memoriam

Although we have many success stories of lives that have been changed and saved through chiropractic care, lifestyle changes, medical science, the elimination of toxins, etc., there is still much work to be done. We have only begun to scratch the surface to understand the deadly combination of various forms of toxins when a person has a suppressed immune system due to a chronic illness. This only intensifies the need for us to continue our research and to strive toward better means of preventing and overcoming chronic illnesses and pain.

This book is dedicated to the memory of my friend Travis Neff, who went home to be with the Lord on January 3, 2016, after a lengthy battle with chronic illness, at the tender age of thirty six. Travis was never able to fulfill his dream of writing a book to encourage people who are battling chronic illness. God had bigger plans for you Travis, serving the Lord in heaven. The apostle Paul wrote in Philippians, "For to me, to live is Christ and to die is gain." We celebrate your life Travis and await for a joyous reunion.

NOTES

Introduction and Chapter 1

1 A. B. Miller, C. Wall, C. J. Baines, P. Sun, T. To, and S. A. Narod, "Twenty five year follow-up for breast cancer incidence and mortality of the Canadian National Breast Screening Study: randomized screening trial." *British Medical Journal* Vol. 348 (2014): g366.

2 Stephen R. Covey, *The Seven Habits of Highly Effective People: Powerful Lessons in Personal Change* (New York: Simon and Schuster, 2004)

3 A. Leaf, "Every Day Is a Gift When You Are over 100." *National Geographic* Vol.143, no.1 (January 1973): 92–119.

Chapter 2

1 http://nationalpainreport.com/the-numbers-game-ii-how-many-americans-have-chronic-pain-8825066.html

2 http://workforce-illness-costs-576b-annually-from-sick-days-to-workers-compensation/#7776e1357256.

3 S. F. Marshal, L. Bernstein, H. Anton-Culver, D. Deapen, Pamela L. Horn-Ross, Ronald K. Ross, and others, "Non-steroidal anti-inflammatory drug use and breast cancer risk by stage and hormone receptor status." *Journal of the National Cancer Institute* Vol.97, no. 11 (June 1, 2005): 805–812.

4 S. Friis, L. Thomassen, H. T. Sørensen, A, Tjønneland, K. Overvad, D. P. Cronin-Fenton, J. H. Olsen, and others, "Nonsteroidal anti-inflammatory drug use and breast cancer risk: a Danish cohort study." *European Journal of Cancer Prev*ention, Vol.17, no. 2 (April 2008): 88–96. doi:10.1097/CEJ.0b013e3282b6fd55.

5 E. S. Schernhammer, J. H. Kang, A. T. Chan, D. S. Michaud, H. G. Skinner, E. Giovannucci, G. A. Colditz, and C. S. Fuchs, "Prospective study of aspirin use

and the risk of pancreatic cancer in women." *Journal of the National Cancer Institute* Vol.96, no. 1 (January 7, 2004): 22–8.

6 A. M. Larson, J. Polson, R. J. Fontana, T. J. Davern, E. Lalani, W. M. Lee, and others, "Acetaminophen-induced acute liver failure: results of a United States multicenter, prospective study." *Hepatology* Vol.42, no. 6 (December 2005): 1364–72.

7 Tim Davern, "The Danger of Mixing Candy and Poison." *San Francisco Chronicle*, August 14, 2004.

8 T. Perenger, P. K. Whelton, and M. J. Klag, "Risk of Kidney Failure with Use of Acetaminophen, Aspirin, and Non-Steroidal Anti-inflammatory Drugs." *New England Journal of Medicine* Vol.331, no. 25 (December 22, 1994): 1675–9.

9 http://www.geoba.se/population.php?pc=world&type=15

10 Adapted from: https://www.cbo.gov/sites/default/files/114th-congress-2015-2016/reports/50724-udEconOutlook.pdf.

11 Paul Zane Pilzner, *The (New) Wellness Revolution* (Hoboken, NJ: John Wiley and Sons, 2007).

12 C. J. Murray, C. Atkinson, K. Bhalla, G. Birbeck, R. Burstein, D. Chou, and others, "The State of US Health, 1990–2010: : Burden of Diseases, Injuries, and Risk Factors." *Journal of the American Medical Association* Vol.310, no. 6 (2013): 591–606.

13 Adapted from:https://www.cancer.gov/about-nci/budget

14 Adapted from:http://jamanetwork.com/journals/jama/article-abstract/2089358

15 A. F. Macedo, I. Douglas, L. Smeeth, H. Forbes, and S. Ebrahim, "Statins and the risk of type 2 diabetes mellitus: cohort study using the UK clinical practice research datalink." *BMC Cardiovascular Disorders,* Vol. 14 (July 15, 2014): 85. doi: 10.1186/1471-2261-14-85.

16 A. L. Culver, I. S. Ockene, R. Balasubramanian, B. C. Olendzki, D. M. Sepavich, Y. Ma, and others, "Statin Use and Risk of Diabetes Mellitus in Postmenopausal Women." *Archives of Internal Medicine* Vol.172, no. 2 (January 23, 2012): 144–152. Epub January 9, 2012. doi: *10.1001/archinternmed.2011.625.*

17 J. G. Salway, *Metabolism at a Glance*, 3rd ed. (Hoboken NJ: Blackwell Publishing, 2004).

18 R. Perkins, University of Southern California, November 2014. Adapted from: https://news.usc.edu/70871/baby-boomers-will-drive-explosion-in-alzheimers-related-costs-in-coming-decades/.

19 J. Glenmullen, *Prozac Backlash: Overcoming the Dangers of Prozac, Zoloft, Paxil, and Other Antidepressants with Safe, Effective Alternatives* (New York: Simon & Schuster, 2001).

20 Marilia Carabotti, et. al, The gut-brain axis: interactions between enteric microbiota, central and enteric nervous systems, *Annals of Gastroenterology,* 28(2): 203–209. Apr-Jun, 2015 PMCID: PMC4367209

21 P. Kidd, Bipolar disorder as cell membrane dysfunction. Progress toward integrative management., *Alternative Medicine Review*, Vol. 9, No. 2, June, 2004,pp 107-135

22 J. J. Cannell, M. Zasloff, C. F. Garland, R. Scragg, and E. Giovannucci, "On the epidemiology of influenza." *Virology Journal* Vol.5 (February 25, 2008): 29. doi: 10.1186/1743-422X-5-29.

23 J. L. Aloia and M. Li-Ng, "Regarding epidemic influenza and vitamin D." *Epidemiology and Infection*, Vol.135, no. 7 (October 2007). doi: http://dx.doi.org/10.1017/S0950268807008308.

24 M. Zasloff, "Fighting Infections with Vitamin D." *Nature Medicine* Vol.12, no. 9 (April 2006): 388–390. doi: 10.1038/nm0406-388.

25 J. Pizzorno, "What we have learned about vitamin D dosing." *Integrative Medicine* Vol.9, no. 1 (February/March 2010).

26 K. L. Munger, S. M. Zhang, E. O'Reilly, M. A. Hernán, M. J. Olek, W. C. Willett, and A. Ascherio, "Vitamin D intake and incidence of multiple sclerosis." *Neurology* Vol.62, no. 1 (January 13, 2004): 60–5.

27 J. J. Cannell, "Autism and Vitamin D." *Medical Hypotheses* Vol.70, no. 4 (2008): 750–9. Epub October 24, 2007.

28 J. Dowd and M. Holick, *The Vitamin D Cure* (Hoboken, NJ: John Wiley and Sons, 2008).

29 G. Schwalfenberg, "Improvement of chronic back pain or failed back surgery with Vitamin D repletion: A case series." *Journal of the American Board of Family Medicine* Vol.22, no. 1 (January-February 2009): 69–74. doi: 10.3122/jabfm.2009.01.080026.

Chapter 3

1 I. H. Page, F. J. Stare, A. C. Corcoran, H. Pollak, and C. F. Wilkinson Jr., "Atherosclerosis and the fat content of the diet." *Circulation* 16 (1957): 164–178.

2 M. S. Donaldson, "Nutrition and cancer: a review of the evidence for an anti-cancer diet." *Nutrition Journal*, no. 3 (October 20, 2004): 19. doi: 10.1186/1475-2891-3-19.

3 R. Blaylock, *Natural Strategies for Cancer Patients,* 1st ed. (New York: Kensington Publishing, 2003).

4 S. Kalmijn, M. P. Van Boxtel, M. Ocké, W. M. Verschuren, D. Kromhout, and L. J. Launer, "Dietary intake of fatty acids and fish in relation to cognitive performance at middle age." Neurology Vol.62, no. 2 (January 27, 2004): 275–80.

5 Ken Midkiff, *The Meat You Eat: How Corporate Farming Has Endangered America's Food Supply.* Reprint ed. (New York: St. Martin's Press, 2005).

6 David Perlmutter, *Grain Brain* (New York: Little, Brown and Company Publishers, 2013).
7 M. M. Kanter, P. M. Kris-Etherton, M. L. Fernandez, K. C. Vickers, and D. L. Katz, "Exploring the Factors that Affect Blood Cholesterol and Heart Disease Risk: Is Dietary Cholesterol as Bad for You as History Leads Us to Believe?" *Advances in Nutrition* Vol.3, no. 5 (September 1, 2012): 711–7. doi: 10.3945/an.111.001321.
8 http://people.uncw.edu/imperialm/UNCW/PLS_506/242516-Heart-Surgeon-Speaks-Out-On-What-Really-Causes-Heart-Disease.pdf
9 S. O. E. Ebbesson, V. S. Venkata, P. B. Higgins, R. R. Fabsitz, L. O. Ebbesson, B. V. Howard, and others, "Fatty acids linked to cardiovascular mortality are associated with risk factors." *International Journal of Circumpolar Health*, Vol.74 (August 12, 2015): 28055. doi: 10.3402/ijch.v74.28055. eCollection 2015.

Chapter 4

1 Bruce Rabin, *Stress Immune Function and Health: The Connection* (New York: Wiley-Liss, 1999)
2 ibid
3 R. Blaylock, *Health and Nutrition Secrets That Can Save Your Life*, revised ed. (Royal Oak, MI: Health Press NA Inc., 2006).
4 K. Cooper, *The Antioxidant Revolution* (Nashville, TN: Thomas Nelson, 1997).
5 M. T. Morter, *Dynamic Health* (Rogers, AR: Best Publishing, 1995).
6 Lawrence Steinman, Elaborate interactions between the immune system and nervous systems, *Nature Immunology*, Vol. 5 May 26, 2004, pp. 575-581

Chapter 5

1 P. Kidd, Bipolar disorder as cell membrane dysfunction. Progress toward integrative management., *Alternative Medicine Review*, Vol. 9, No. 2, June, 2004,pp 107-135
2 S.M. O'Mahony, Serotonin, tryptophan metabolism and the brain-gut-microbiome axis, *Behavioural Brain Research*,Vol. 277, 15 January 2015, Pages 32–48,
3 L. E. Hebert, P. A. Scherr, J. L. Bienias, D. A. Bennett, and D. A. Evans, "State Specific Projections of Alzheimer's Disease Prevalence through 2025." *Neurology* Vol.62, no. 9 (May 11, 2004): 1645.
4 J. Salway, *Metabolism at a Glance, pg. 52*
5 M. Studer, M. Briel, B. Leimenstoll, T. R. Glass, and H. C. Bucher, "Effect of different anti-lipidemic agents and diets on mortality: a systematic review." *Archives of Internal Medicine* Vol.165, no. 7 (April 11, 2005): 725–30.

6 L. Vanderhaeghe and K. Kasrst, *Healthy Fats for Life: Preventing and Treating Common Health Problems with Essential Fatty Acids*, 1st ed. (John Wiley & Sons, 2004).

7 L. K. Saugstad, "Are neurodegenerative disorder and psychotic manifestations avoidable brain dysfunctions with adequate dietary omega-3?" *Nutrition and Health* Vol.18, no. 2 (2006): 89–101.

8 M. V. Boswell, ed., *Weiner's Pain Management: A Practical Guide for Clinicians*, 7th ed. (Boca Raton, FL: CRC Press, 2005), 584–5.

9 Ridker, P.M., et.al, Comparison of c- reactive protein and low density lipoprotein cholesterol levels in the prediction of first cardiovascular events, *New England Journal of Medicine*, Vol. 347 (20) November 14, 2002, pp1557-1565

10 Yu-Wei Roy Chen, J. M. Leung, and D. D. Sin, "A systematic review of diagnostic biomarkers of COPD exacerbation." *PLoS One*_Vol.11, no. 7 (July 19, 2016): e0158843. doi: 10.1371/journal.pone.0158843. eCollection 2016.

11 L. Yang, Z. Song, W. Cao, Y. Wang, H. Lu, G. Sun, et. al, "Effects of diets with different n-6/n-3 fatty acids on cardiovascular risk factors in mice fed high-fat diets." *Wei Sheng Yan Jiu* Vol.45, no. 3 (May 2016): 436–41.

12 Schnyder, G., et.al, Effect of homocysteine-lowering therapy with folic acid, vitamin B12 and Vitamin B6 on clinical outcome after percutaneous coronary intervention: A randomized controlled trial, *Journal of the American Medical Association*, Vol. 288;(8), August 28, 2002, pp. 973-979

13 S. R. Mirhafez, M. Ebrahimi, M. Saberi Karimian, A. Avan, M. Tayefi, M. Ghayour-Mobarhan, and others, "Serum high-sensitivity C-reactive protein as a biomarker in patients with metabolic syndrome: evidence-based study with 7284 subjects." *European Journal of Clinical Nutrition*, July 27, 2016. Epub ahead of print. doi: 10.1038/ejcn.2016.111.

14 R. Marcelino, J. Oliva García, J. J. Alemán Sánchez, D. Almeida González, S. Domínguez Coello, A. Cabrera de León, and others, "Lipid and inflammatory biomarker profiles in early insulin resistance." *Acta Diabetol* (July 18, 2016). Epub ahead of print. doi: 10.1007/s00592-016-0885-6.

15 Barry Sears, *The Omega Rx Zone*, 1st ed. (William Morrow, 2002).

16 Barry Sears, *Toxic Fat* (Thomas Nelson Press, 2008).

17 M. Boswell, *Weiner's Pain Management*, 584–85.

Chapter 6

1 Sears, *Toxic Fat.*

2 Boswell, *Weiner's Pain Management*, 584–85.

3 K. Singh, *Oxidative Stress, Disease and Cancer* (Imperial College Press, 2006).

4 S. Miwa, *Oxidative Stress in Aging: From Model Systems to Human Diseases* (Humana Press, 2008).

5 M. Newport, *Alzheimer's Disease: What If There Was a Cure. The Story of Ketones*, 2nd ed. (Basic Health Publications, 2013).
6 D. Perlmutter, *The Better Brain Book* (Riverhead Books, 2004), 21–3.
7 R.Blaylock, *Health and Nutrition Secrets: That can save your life*
8 A. L. Hansen, K. Wijndaele, N. Owen, D. J. Magliano, A. A. Thorp, J. E. Shaw, and D. W. Dunstan, "Adverse associations of increases in television viewing time with 5-year changes in glucose homoeostasis markers: the Aus diab study." *Diabetic Medicine* Vol.29, no. 7 (July 2012): 918–25. doi: 10.1111/j.1464-5491.2012.03656.
9 D. A. Christakis, F. J. Zimmerman, D. L. DiGiuseppe, and C. A. McCarty, "Early television exposure and subsequent attentional problems in children." *Pediatrics* Vol.113, no. 4 (April 2004).

Chapter 7

1 J. Uribarri, S. Woodruff, S. Goodman, W. Cai, X. Chen, R. Pyzik, and others, "Advanced glycation end products in foods and a practical guide to the reduction in the diet." *Journal of the American Dietetic Association* 110, no. 9 (June 2010): 911–16.
2 K. E. Davis, C. Prasad, P. Vijayagopal, S. Juma, and V. Simrhan, "Advanced glycation end products, inflammation, and chronic metabolic diseases: links in a chain?" *Critical Reviews in Food Science and Nutrition* Vol.56, no. 6 (April 25, 2016): 989–98. doi: 10.1080/10408398.2012.744738.
3 M. Takeuchi, S. Kikuchi, N. Sasaki, T. Suzuki, T. Watai, S. Yamagishi, and others, "Involvement of advanced glycation end products in Alzheimer's disease." *Current Alzheimer Research* Vol.1, no. 1 (February 2004): 39–46.
4 A. Machado-Lima, R. T. Iborra, R. S. Pinto, G. Castilho, C. H. Sartori, M. Passarelli, and others, "In type 2 diabetes mellitus glycated albumin alters macrophage gene expression impairing ABCA1-mediated cholesterol efflux." *Journal of Cell Physiology* Vol.230, no. 6 (June 2015): 1250–7. doi: 10.1002/jcp.24860.
5 M. W. Poulsen, R. V. Hedegaard, J. M. Andersen, B. de Courten, S. Büge, L. O. Dragsted, and others, "Advanced glycation end products in food and their effects on health." *Food and Chemical Toxicology* Vol.60 (October 2013): 10–37. Epub July 16, 2013. doi: 10.1016/j.fct.2013.06.052.
6 A. P. S. Kong and J. C. N. Chan, "Cancer risk in type 2 diabetes." *Current Diabetes Reports* Vol.12 (2012): 325. doi:10.1007/s11892-012-0277-4.
7 K. B. Michels, B. A. Rosner, W. C. Chumlea, G. A. Colditz, and W. C. Willett, "Preschool diet and adult risk of breast cancer." *International Journal of Cancer* 118, no. 3 (February 2006): 749–54. doi: 10.1002/ijc.21407.

8 R. J. Klement and U. Kämmerer, "Is there a role for carbohydrate restriction in the treatment and prevention of cancer?" *Nutrition and Metabolism* Vol.8 (October 2011): 75. doi: 10.1186/1743-7075-8-75.

9 Adapted from: http://articles.mercola.com/sites/articles/archive/2009/09/05/another-poison-hiding-in-your-environment.aspx; Bromines: Avoid This if You Want to Keep Your Thyroid Healthy, *Mercola.com*; September 05, 2009.

10 L. R. Howe, "Inflammation and breast cancer: Cyclooxygenase/prostaglandin signaling and breast cancer." *Breast Cancer Research* Vol.9 (2007): 210. doi: 10.1186/bcr1678.

11 R. Ness and J. A. Cauley, "Antibiotics and breast cancer—what is the meaning of this?" *Journal of the American Medical Association* Vol.291, no. 7 (February 2004): 880–81. doi: 10.1001/jama.291.7.880.

12 C. M. Velicer, S. R. Heckbert, J. W. Lampe, J. D. Potter, C. A. Robertson, and S. H. Taplin, "Antibiotic use in relation to the risk of breast cancer." *Journal of the American Medical Association* Vol.291, no. 7 (February 2004): 827–35.

13 K. M. Steele, J. E. Carreiro, J. H. Viola, J. A. Conte, and L. C. Ridpath, "Effect of osteopathic manipulative treatment on middle ear effusion following acute otitis media in young children: a pilot study." *Journal of the American Osteopathic Association* Vol.114, no. 6 (June 2014): 436–47. doi: 10.7556/jaoa.2014.094.

Chapter 8

1 A. J. Baker, R. J. Moulton, V. H. MacMillan, and P. M. Shedden, "Excitatory amino acids in cerebrospinal fluid following traumatic brain injury in humans." *Journal of Neurosurgery* 79, no. 3 (September 1993): 369–72.

2 A. Doble, "The role of excitotoxicity in neurodegenerative disease: implications for therapy." *Pharmacology and Therapeutics* 81, no. 3 (March 1999): 163–221.

3 G. Schwartz, *In Bad Taste: The MSG Symptom Complex*, revised ed. (Santa Fe, NM: Health Press, 1999).

4 J. D. Smith, C. M. Terpening, S. O. Schmidt, and J. G. Gums, "Relief of fibromyalgia symptoms following discontinuation of dietary excitotoxins." *Annals of Pharmacotherapy* Vol.35, no. 6 (June 2001): 702–6.

5 Adapted from: http://www.sfgate.com/health/article/Study-Chemicals-pollutants-found-in-newborns-3207709.php; December 2009.

6 Neil Miller and G. S. Goldman, "Infant mortality rates regressed against number of vaccine doses routinely given: Is there a biochemical or synergistic toxicity?" *Human & Experimental Toxicology* Vol.30, no. 9 (September 2011): 1420–28. doi: 10.1177/0960327111407644.

7 https://vaers.hhs.gov/data/data

8 A.S. Holmes, et.al, Reduced levels of mercury in first baby haircuts of autistic children, *International Journal of Toxicology*, Vol 22, No. 4, July-Aug 2003, pp277-285

9 S. Seneff, R. M. Davidson, and Liu Jingjing, "Empirical data confirms autism symptoms related to aluminum and acetaminophen exposure." *Entropy* Vol.14, no. 11 (2012): 2227–53. doi: 10.3390/e14112227.

10 P. J. Landrigan, "What Causes Autism: Exploring the Environmental Contribution." *Current Opinion Pediatrics* Vol.22, no. 2 (April 2010): 219–25. doi: 10.1097/MOP.0b013e328336eb9a.

11 M. Kogan, S. J. Blumberg, L. A. Scheive, C. A. Boyle, J. M. Perrin, P. C. Van Dyke, and others, "Prevalence of parent reported diagnosis of autism among children in the US, 2007." *Pediatrics* Vol.124, no. 5 (November 2009).

12 O. Strannegard and I. L. Strannegård, "The causes of increasing prevalence of allergy: Is atopy a microbial depravation disorder?" *Allergy* Vol.56, no. 2 (February 2001): 91–102.

13 I. J. Elenkov, R. L. Wilder, G. P. Chrousos, and E. S. Vizi, "The sympathetic nerve: An integrative interface between two super systems. The brain and immune system." *Pharmacological Reviews* Vol.52, no. 4 (December 2000): 595–638.

14 R A Hites, et.al, Global assessment of organic contaminants in farmed salmon, *Science*, Vol.303, No.5655, pp. 226-229

15 Ken Midkiff, *The Meat You Eat: How Corporate Farming Has Endangered America's Food Supply*

16 R. A. Hites, J. A. Foran, S. J. Schwager, B. A. Knuth, M. C. Hamilton, and D. O. Carpenter, "Global Assessment of Poly Brominated Diphenyl Ethers in Farmed and Wild Salmon." *Environmental Science and Technology* Vol.38, no. 19 (October 1, 2004): 4945–9.

17 ibid

18 Ken Midkiff, *The Meat You Eat: How Corporate Farming Has Endangered America's Food Supply*

19 ibid

20 J. F. Wilson, "Balancing the Risk and Benefits of Fish Consumption." *Annals of Internal Medicine* Vol.141, no. 12 (2004): 977–980. doi: 10.7326/0003-4819-141-12-200412210-00024.

21 Kelly Weaver, et.al, The content of unfavorable fatty acids found in commonly eaten fish, *Journal of the American Dietetic Association*, Vol. 108 no.7 July 2008, pp.1/178- 1185

22 https://public.health.oregon.gov/HealthyEnvironments Recreation/FishConsumption/Documents/fishscreeninglevels.pdf

23 J. F. Wilson, "Balancing the Risk and Benefits of Fish Consumption."

24 http://www.washingtonpost.com/wp-dyn/content/article/2009/01/26/AR2009012601831.html

25 W. Davis, *Wheat Belly: Lose the Wheat, Lose the Weight, and Find Your Path Back to Health*, reprint ed. (Rodale Books, 2014).

26 J. Braley and R. Hoggan, *Dangerous Grains; Why Gluten Cereal Grains May Be Hazardous to Your Health* (Avery Press, 2002).

27 B. Smith, *The Emergence of Agriculture*. no. 54 of the Scientific American Library series,1998.

28 Z. Honeycutt, adapted from http://www.momsacrossamerica.com/ stunning corn comparison: gmo versus non gmo; MomsAcrossAmerica.com, March 15, 2013.

29 A. Samsel and S. Seneff, "Glyphosate's suppression of cytochrome P450 enzymes and amino acid biosynthesis by the gut microbiome: Pathways to modern diseases." *Entropy* Vol.15, no. 4 (2013): 1416–63. doi: 10.3390/e15041416.

Chapter 9

1 B. Yang, S. Fan, X. Zhi, D. Wang, Y. Li, G. Sun, and others, "Associations of MTHFR C677T and MTRR A66G gene polymorphisms with metabolic syndrome: a case-control study in Northern China." *International Journal of Molecular Sciences* Vol.15, no. 12 (November 25, 2014): 21687–702. doi: 10.3390/ijms151221687.

2 R. J. Schmidt, R. L. Hansen, J. Hartiala, H. Allayee, L. C. Schmidt, I. Hertz-Picciotto, and others, "Prenatal vitamins, one carbon metabolism gene variants, and risk for autism." *Epidemiology* Vol.22, no. 4 (July 2011): 476–85. doi: 10.1097/EDE.0b013e31821d0e30.

3 N. Stewart (October 30, 2014) adapted from: http://www.crnusa.org/prpdfs/CRNPR14-CRNCCSurvey103014.pdf.

4 D. R. Davis, M. D. Epp, and H. D. Riordan, "Changes in USDA food composition data for 43 garden crops, 1950 to 1999." *Journal of the American College of Nutrition* Vol.23, no. 6 (December 2004): 669–82.

5 S. Schwab, A. Zierer, A. Schneider, M. Heier, W. Koenig, B. Thorand, and others, "Vitamin E supplementation is associated with lower levels of C-reactive protein only in higher dosages and combined with other antioxidants: The Cooperative Health Research in the Region of Augsburg (KORA) F4 study." *British Journal of Nutrition* Vol.113, no. 11 (June 14, 2015): 1782–91. Epub April 21, 2015. doi: 10.1017/S0007114515000902.

6 Lora Vanderhaeghe, Karlene Kasrst, *Healthy Fats for Life: Preventing and Treating Common Health Problems With Essential Fatty Acids* (Hoboken,NJ: Wiley and Sons, 2004) pg.185

7 J. Gutman, *Glutathione: Your Key to Health* (Kudo.ca Communications, 2008).

8 G. J. Brewer, "Risk of copper toxicity contributing to cognitive decline in the aging population and to Alzheimer's disease." *Journal of the American College of Nutrition* Vol.28, no. 3 (June 2009): 238–42.
9 N. López, C. Tormo, I. De Blas, I. Llinares, and J. Alom, "Oxidative stress and Alzheimer's disease and mild cognitive impairment." *Journal of Alzheimer's Disease* Vol.33, no. 3 (2013): 823–9. doi: 10.3233/JAD-2012-121528.
10 Q. Xu, C. G. Parks, L. A. DeRoo, R. M. Cawthon, D. P. Sandler, and H. Chen, "Multivitamin use and telomere length in women." *American Journal of Clinical Nutrition* Vol.89, no. 6 (June 2009): 1857–63. Epub March 11, 2009. doi: 10.3945/ajcn.2008.26986.

Chapter 10

1 Adapted from http://www.vivo.colostate.edu/hbooks/pathphys/misc_topics/radicals.html.
2 N. Panth, K. R. Paudel, and K. Parajuli, "Reactive Oxygen Species: A Key Hallmark of Cardiovascular Disease." *Advances in Medicine* 2016 (2016): 9152732. Epub September 28, 2016. doi: 10.1155/2016/9152732.
3 H. Ahsan, A. Ali, and R. Ali, "Oxygen free radicals and systemic autoimmunity." *Clinical and Experimental Immunology* 131, no. 3 (March 2003): 398–404. doi: 10.1046/j.1365-2249.2003.02104.x.
4 M. T. Morter, *An Apple a Day? Is It Enough Today?* (BEST Research Inc., 1996).
5 M. S. Donaldson, "Nutrition and cancer: a review of the evidence for an anti-cancer diet." *Nutrition Journal* Vol.3 (October 20, 2004): 19. doi: 10.1186/1475-2891-3-19.
6 S. A. Johnson and B. H. Arjmandi, "Evidence for anti-cancer properties of blueberries: a mini-review." *Anti-Cancer Agents in Medicinal Chemistry* Vol.13, no. 8 (October 2013): 1142–8.
7 E. P. Cherniack, "A berry thought-provoking idea: the potential role of plant polyphenols in the treatment of age-related cognitive disorders." *British Journal of Nutrition* Vol.108, no. 5 (September 2012): 794–800. Epub April 5, 2012. doi: 10.1017/S0007114512000669.
8 M. Mahesh, M. Bharathi, M. Raja Gopal Reddy, P. Pappu, U. K. Putcha, S. M. Jeyakumar, and others, "Carrot juice ingestion attenuates high fructose-induced circulatory pro-inflammatory mediators in weanling Wistar rats." *Journal of the Science of Food and Agriculture* (July 15, 2016). Epub ahead of print. doi: 10.1002/jsfa.7906.
9 Y. Tantamango-Bartley, K. Jaceldo-Siegl, J. Fan, and G. Fraser, "Vegetarian diets and the incidence of cancer in a low-risk population." *Cancer Epidemiology Biomarkers and Prevention* Vol.22, no. 2 (February 2013): 286–94. Epub November 20, 2012. doi: 10.1158/1055-9965.EPI-12-1060.

10 M. Mouria, A. S. Gukovskaya, Y. Jung, P. Buechler, O. Hines, S. J. Pandol, and others, "Food-derived polyphenols inhibit pancreatic cancer growth through mitochondrial cytochrome C release and apoptosis." *International Journal of Cancer* Vol.98, no. 5 (April 10, 2002): 761–69. doi: 10.1002/ijc.10202.
11 http://articles.mercola.com/sites/articles/archive/2015/04/29/junk-food-metabolism.aspx
12 ibid, Kelly Weaver, et.al, The content of unfavorable fatty acids found in commonly eaten fish

Chapter 11

1 F.Carrick, Changes in brain function after manipulation of the cervical spine, *Journal of Manipulative and Physiological Therapeutics*. Vol. 8, Oct. 20, 1997; 529–545.
2 M.Driscoll, et.al. Effects of spinal manipulative therapy on autonomic activity and the cardiovascular system: a case study using the electrocardiogram and arterial tonometry, *Journal of Manipulative and Physiological Therapeutics*, Vol.23, No.8, 2000; 545–550

www.ingramcontent.com/pod-product-compliance
Lightning Source LLC
Chambersburg PA
CBHW020511290526
45786CB00002B/556

* 9 7 8 1 5 1 2 7 8 6 4 1 5 *